The Science of
Homoeopathic Immunology

Pharmacodynamics of Homoeopathic
Medicines Explained

JOHN MICHEL WARNER

First Edition

Vainskull Publication, Madagaskar

First Edition: 2019

All rights are reserved. No part of this publication may be reproduced, stored in a retrieval system or transmitted, in any form or any means, mechanical, photocopying, recording or otherwise, without prior written permission of the publishers.

Price: $14 (Fourteen dollar only)

© Copyright with the Publisher

Published by:

J M Warner
for
VainSkull Publishers Ltd
Skull Island, Madagaskar.
Email: jmwarnerx@gmail.com

ISBN:

DEDICATION

If you feel like praying for me, pray to Him who is endowed with the following virtues:

1. He must be the One and only one
2. He must be the absolute
3. Nobody gave birth to Him, neither He gave birth to anybody
4. Nothing in the universe resembles to Him
5. He does not want food, but likes food given to them who want it
6. He is powerful but loathes power which falls upon the powerless

Let's start our journey in search of such:

One

CONTENTS

	Acknowledgments	i
	Preface to the First Edition	3
1	Farrington's Dream: Plausibility of a Scientific Explanation	5
2	Definition of Disease and Man from Modern Biological Perspective	10
3	Hahnemann's *miasm* and *Vital force*: Equivalent to Medieval Miasma Theory and "Vitalism"?	29
4	Hahnemann's Disease-agent Equivalent to Germs?	45
5	Homoeopathy: an Overnight Discovery? How much credible is the story of cinchona?	56
6	Hahnemann's Postulation and Warner's *Momentum*	67
7	Mechanism-of-Action of Homoeopathic Medicines and Warner's *Momentum*	73
8	Effective Sites of Administration of Homoeopathic Medicines	93
9	Outline of a Homoeopathic Materia Medica: How we should read medicines?	102
10	Exploration of Therapeutics of Arnica Mont in terms of Hahnemann's Postulation	110
11	Succussion and High Potency: Century-old Injustice Done to Hahnemann	118
12	Bibliography	128

ACKNOWLEDGMENTS

I would like to express my thanks of gratitude to all those homeopaths and authors who spent their lives in researching and discovering the scientific features of homeopathy for years. Furthermore, I am greatly indebted to my father who taught me not to compromise the truth in any situation. I am sorry, I failed.

PREFACE TO THE FIRST EDITION

It was almost fifteen years ago. One day a client requested me to write on the quackery (?) of Homoeopathy. It was an eight-page paper which was of 40 dollar worth. I needed the money very much; so I started searching on the internet for articles which argue against Homoeopathy. I wrote the paper; the client happily paid me the money. But I was not satisfied. There was something disturbing in the paper I wrote for my client. The points on which I argued against Homeopathy never won my heart. Even more disturbing was my reading of the 6th edition of Hahnemann's *Organon of Medicine*. The philosophy of the *man* with its complex self-defense functionalities was not easy for me to comprehend. Neither had I had any strong ground to oppose against Hahnemann's philosophical concepts such as *suppression*, merits and demerits of *suppuration*, autonomous and self-defending *vital force* and many others. Before I wrote the paid article on Homoeopathy, I had written many articles on the immune system of human body for my clients. So, there was a doubt in the remote corner of my mind that somehow Hahnemann stole the concept of *vital force* from Metchnikoff, Louis Pasteur, Jenner, etc. But strikingly I noticed that both Elie Metchnikoff and Louis Pasteur were born several years after Hahnemann's death. Furthermore, I noticed that there is not even a single article on the internet which attempts to falsify the philosophical tenets of Hahnemann's *Organon*. Rather those criticisms against Homoeopathy mainly revolve around two basic claims:

a. That is, Hahnemann's concepts i.e. *miasm* and *vital force* are medieval and, therefore, outdated.

b. That is, Homoeopathic potencies do not contain any medicine (so they are mere placeboes).

Regarding the first point I felt that that those authors have never read the *Organon of Medicine* carefully. So, very regretfully they failed to perceive the new connotations which Hahnemann wanted to convey in those conventional words, *miasm and vital force*. They confuse Hahnemann's *miasm* and *vital force* with medieval '*Miasma Theory*' and '*Vitalism*'. Even more regretfully almost all of the homeopaths excluding the few exceptions perceive Hahnemann's *miasm and vital force* as the medieval ones. Regarding the second claim, I felt that Hahnemann uses high dilution in the mid of his career as a homoeopathic doctor when he was go through extensive research and experimentation. But during the final years of his life he decisively avoided the use of potencies higher than the 30th centesimal. Also if he were aware of the Avogadro Limit, he would decide differently on the high ultra dilution.

However, in this book, I have tried to uphold all the philosophical tenets and practices of Homeopathy from a modern biological view. In doing so, I further felt that Homoeopathy is the result of Hahnemann's opposition against the traditional quackery in the name of scientific treatment. He vehemently opposed *Suppression* (a unique connotation for his contemporary scholars) about 250 years ago. But even during these days, this quackery of suppressive treatment is occurring with modern medical practices of using painkillers, biological function suppressor, etc. I feel that Hahnemann should be awarded the Nobel Prize posthumously for his work on immune system (vital power) and homoeopathy. Do you agree with me?

J. M. Warner
2019-10-09
Skull Island, Madagskar

1
FARRINGTON'S DREAM: PLAUSIBILITY OF A SCIENTIFIC EXPLANATION OF HOMOEOPATHY

In his book, A *Supplement to Gross' Comparative Materia Medica*, E A Farrington claimed, "Our *Materia Medica* is a natural science, the Future must prove it."[1] He dreamt that homoeopathic concepts and findings would be proved in the laboratory. Who will materialize this dream? Who will prove the scientific basis of Homeopathy? Materialization of Farrington's dream (that is, "Future science must be able to explain the truth of Homoeopathy") is far-fetched because of the animosity of the multibillion-dollar drug industry owners. It is quite reasonable that they will feel the terror when they see that a single pill (which costs almost nothing) relieves the patient of the incurable disease which seems to be the worst nightmare for the Allopaths. The Future of their "multibillion-dollar business" is quite obvious. That is, the small, dwarfish and negligible pills are supposed to destroy their "moneymaking machines" with merciless integrity. So, it is quite expected that they will turn their back on the reality of homoeopathy. But being the successors of Hahnemann, S T Kent, Farrington, etc, we, in the 21st century, urgently need a theoretical and scientific explanation of what we do, why we did and how our medicines work.

We have innumerous examples of the cure of apparently incurable diseases where the Allopaths failed in some ways or others. Those are the cases where the Allopaths' only option is their surgical knighthood or their lifelong medication (palliative treatment). Millions of patients around the world will testify the efficacy of Homoeopathic medicines. Indeed, despite the overwhelming antagonism of Allopaths, Homoeopathy had survived on the solace and satisfaction of these patients during the last two centuries after

---

[1] E A Farrington. *A Supplement to Gross' Comparative Materia Medica*. Volume 1.

Homoeopathy began its journey. Like the past, Homoeopathy will continue to score success in treating more and more patients. But why will not the modern scholars acknowledge the efficacy of Homoeopathic medicines? Why don't they see that a patient with several tumors or cysts in her uterus or his neck once ran away from the surgeons' knives took refuge to a homoeopath's age-worn table. When he/she was talking to that homoeopath, she was quite hysterical. Now she was laughing while telling her happy memories with her beloved husband. But right then she was crying out of severe despair that she will never be a mother because you, the allopaths, advised her to cut off her uterus. She could not sleep for years. She suffered from metrorrhagia for several months. Severe pain does not allow her to stay at rest even for an hour. That homoeopath prescribed few pills of Pulsatilla 30 everyday for thirty days. After one month the patient reported that her pain was gone and now she slept quite well; but still her name was irregular and scanty. But she was quite confident that the cysts in her uterus could be cured. Later, Bacilinum 30/Calc Phos 30/ Aurum M Nat 30 cured her metrorrhagia and most of the cysts were gone. Finally, she became the mother of four babies. Almost every homoeopath, around the world, has some stories of such legendary cures to tell you. If you do not believe in these stories, why don't you investigate into these claims of cures yourselves?

WHY THIS VOID OF A SCIENTIFIC THEORIZATION OF HOMOEOPATHY?

Now, the question is what Pulsatilla/Calc.Phos/Bacilinum/AurumM.N did to that patient's uterus? Indeed, pharmacodynamics and pharmacokinetics of almost every Homoeopathic medicine is still unexplored. Why unexplored? Our observation and data fairly show that treating a patient according to Hahnemann's philosophy, "like cure like" most often results into stunning examples of cure. When Hahnemann, in the first half of the 18th century, declared that "Treat the patient (man), not the disease (not its symptoms)", it was really difficult for the medical frontiers of the time to understand what Hahnemann wanted to mean by the term, 'man' or '*vital force*'. Also it was confusing for them to comprehend the role of the 'man' in curing a disease because Hahnemann's contemporary medical science did not know much about the 'man' or 'vital power' or the 'immune system'. Indeed, scientists started to pay more attention to the 'man' or the "man's power to defend against disease" or 'vital power' or 'immune system' during the first half of the 20th century with Ilya Ilyich Metchnikoff's discovery of phagocyte cells. Metchnikoff was awarded Nobel Prize for his experiment in which he pushed some citrus thorns into starfish larvae and observed that some cells gathered around that foreign body and came to the conclusion that any living being's immune system produces phagocytes to defend against the foreign body.[2]

---

[2] Wikipedia. "Élie Metchnikoff", https://en.wikipedia.org/wiki/Élie_Metchnikoff

Here, note that Hahnemann, long before Metchnikoff's discovery of 'phagocyte', advocated the concept of the "man's ability to defend against any disease agent".[3] Obviously Hahnemann expressed the abstract essence of this ability of the man's immune power to defend against diseases in such an era when people did not know much about the germs until Louis Pasteur's discovery.

It is very much expected that Hahnemann could not use any modern immunological terminologies to describe man's ability to defend itself from external organisms and forces, because modern immunology started its journey with Metchnikoff's discovery of phagocytes in 1882 long after Hahnemann's death. But he was quite aware of this ability of human body. In many lines of the *Organon of Medicine*, he attempted to provide an outline of this self-protecting power of human body. For him, this power is the "spirit-like *vital force* (dynamis)" or "the reasoning spirit" or "self-sustaining spirit-like *vital force*" which "animates the material human organism" (regulation of immune organs), "reigns in supreme sovereignty" (super intelligent defending immune system), "maintains the sensations and activities of all the parts of the living organism in a harmony" (sensory nervous functions, the regulatory control of Central Nervous System on the whole), etc.[4] He generalized all of these functions as *vital functions* which are necessary to keep a man healthy. He knew nothing about the modern biological discoveries on the nervous system; but he advocated that one of the functions of the *vital force* is to "feel, or act, or maintain itself". Read between the lines from the *Organon of Medicine*:

> In the state of health the spirit-like *vital force* (dynamis) animates the material human organism reigns in supreme sovereignty. It maintains the sensations and activities of all the parts of the living organism in a harmony that obliges wonderment. The reasoning spirit who inhabits the organism can thus freely use this healthy living instrument to reach the lofty goal of human existence. (Organon of Medicine, Para-9)[5]

> Without the *vital force* the material organism is unable to feel, or act, or maintain itself....Only because of the immaterial being (vital principle, *vital force*) that animates it in health and in disease can it feel and maintain its vital functions. (Organon of Medicine, Para-10)[6]

So for Hahnemann, symptoms of disease are essentially the language of the "disturbed *vital force*", a physical state in which the "disturbed *vital force*"

---

[3] The whole phrase "man's ability to defend against any *disease agent*" is indeed the essence of Hahnemann's concept of *spirit like* v*ital force* in the Organon of Medicine

[4] Samuel Hahneman, Organon of Medicine, Para-6 to para 10

[5] Samuel Hahneman, Organon of Medicine, Para-9

[6] Samuel Hahneman, Organon of Medicine, Para-10

fights against the disturbance, as he says in para-7 of the *Organon of Medicine*, "One may know a disease only by its symptoms....So it is the totality of symptoms, *the outer image expressing the inner essence of the disease, i.e., of the disturbed vital force*".[7] According to this new way of viewing disease, Hahnemann advocates that *suppuration* (also skin eruptions) is one of the many symptoms which are caused by the body's *vital functions* against disturbance in *vital force*. In a similar fashion, modern immunology also considers "suppuration" as a part of the man's defenses against the hostile presence in the body. So, he advocated that 'suppuration' is not the disease because it is merely the response of the man against the hostile force present in the organism. So it may be confusing in apparent eyes to emphasize, going against the traditional reasoning, that the 'suppuration' (or skin eruption) of the 'man' should not be obstructed (or wiped out) by any external application such as surgery, ointment, scorching, etc. Here please note that Hahnemann's 'suppuration (or skin eruption) as a part of the man's defense against the foreign body (*disease agent*)' is quite equivalent to modern 'immunological response to foreign body'. After about 250 years, our knowledge of modern immunology helps us to understand Hahnemann's complex thoughts as the philosophic abstractions of modern concepts of immune system; but was it easy for his contemporary scholars to do so? Nope! The mainstream medical society continued their antagonism against Hahnemann. He was banished from his country for his thoughts.

The distance between Homoeopathy and modern medical science began to grow firstly because Hahnemann's contemporary medical scholars failed to understand the apparently confusing abstraction of the '*man*' or '*immune power*' due to their own limitations and secondly, because the Homoeopaths themselves failed to explain their practice from the scientific viewpoint. Homeopathy went on its own way without making any effort to explain its concepts in the light of modern medical science because Homeopaths were self-satisfied with thousands of evidences of cures. Here, homoeopaths made two mistakes: first, they failed to differentiate between medical science and medical practices; second, because of this failure, they started criticizing their contemporary medical practices and the medical science as well. (Criticisms against such medical practices were quite justified; criticizing and ignoring the scientific findings have, so far, proved to be quite detrimental). On the contrary, the emerging medical researchers started loathing Homoeopathy partly because they could not find the '*man*' (or the role of the *man* in defending itself from external harmful influence) and mostly because homoeopathic pills proved to be quite detrimental to the dream, pride and vanity of their colossal operation theatre and machines. Now, it is time to bridge the gap. However, modern medical science began to know the "Man" more and more but in different name. They called it "Immune system". They

---

[7] Samuel Hahneman, Organon of Medicine, Para-7

learnt that:

> It is the *immune system* that protects a man from diseases. If it is weak, man frequently becomes prone to illness. Different man inherits different degrees of *immune strength* by birth. Men's *immune system* may be weakened by various unhealthy life style and activities.[8]

Quite amazingly Hahnemann preached the concept two centuries ago and faced overwhelming animosity of the so-called medical frontiers. For clarification, let's replace the tern, 'immune system' with Hahnemann's term '*vital force*':

> It is the *vital force* that protects a man from diseases. If it is weak, man frequently becomes prone to illness. Different man inherits different degrees of *vital force* by birth. Men's *vital force* may be weakened by various unhealthy life style and activities.[9]

Hahnemann finally concluded that when a man is ill, it is the *man* (or the *vital force/immune system*) which is sick. So, he concluded, "treat the *man*, not the *disease*". Such claim of Hahnemann was even more confusing for the people of the 18th century who knew nothing about the *man* or the *vital force* (immune system). But now-a-days it is easier to understand Hahnemann's claim, because scientists know more about the complex functions and nature of the '*man*' or '*immune system*'. So, Homoeopathy needs modern medical knowledge more than ever and than other pathies needs it in the 21st century. Since observations show that homoeopathic medicines can cure, we must use modern medical theories to explain these medicines. In this article, we will try to explain Homoeopathy medicines in the light of modern medical theories. But prior to it, we try to explain the basic philosophical concepts of Homoeopathy in contrary to conventional medical practices. Homoeopathy is the only therapeutic strategy which is well-equipped with self-explanatory philosophical concepts which are quite able to challenge the validity of the conventional medical practices. How? Let's examine the philosophical concepts in comparison to those of Allopathic practices side by side. Then you yourself will judge the validity of the philosophical trends of the two treatment methods.

---

[8] It is the gist of what scientists and researchers consider the immune system.
[9] It is indeed the gist of what Hahnemann says about the *Vital force* in the Organon of Medicine

2
DEFINITION OF *DISEASE* AND *MAN* FROM MODERN BIOLOGICAL PERSPECTIVE

Homoeopathy began its journey during the ripe stage of Enlightenment in the late 18th century. During this period, reasons began to dominate the traditional beliefs and superstitions about the reality. John Dalton proposed his Atomic Theory and laid the basis of Modern Physics and Chemistry during this era.. Later, his successors developed and corrected it in order to give birth to a more accurate one. During this period, Hahnemann proposed his contemporary world to view the 'man' as 'the autocratic and dynamic defense' or 'vital power' against ailment. So, physicians should treat the 'man', not the disease. It was too modern and real an assumption to be acknowledged by his contemporary Rationalists. Hahnemann's proposition was clearly a threat against the dominating medical belief. How the existing rationalism tends to defy Hahnemann's assumption is shown in the following discussion.

Hahnemann's concept of the 'Man' (or 'Vitale' or Immune System), as the autocratic and dynamic defense against diseases, has always challenged the traditional physicians' heroic hegemony over a patient's pathogenic condition. The core sentiment which shaped the traditionalist treatment process is mercilessly a heroic one: "If the boil is disturbing the man, blow it with merciless triumph". Look how this heroism over the pathogens has evolved along a period of past 200 years. Pre-Pasteurian physicians would suggest that "if the boil is disturbing the man, blow it with merciless triumph". Later, after Luis Pasture's discovery of germs as the pathogens, they began to suggest that "Kill the germs which cause the boils". But simultaneously with the discovery of antibiotics, modern science further discovered how affected cells of human organs produce inflammatory Interferonal Cytokines. So, they began to use antibiotics along with anti-inflammatory and immunosuppressive NSAID drugs without giving a second thought to the ramifications caused by them. Obviously, they did not need to pay attention to the ramifications of these drugs, the vast majority of commoners, remaining oblivious to those ramifications, were ready to pay vast wealth and money to those physicians in order to be cured quickly by those immunosuppressive medicines.

Opposing this traditional attempt to cure the symptoms or diseases with immunosuppressive medicines, Hahnemann suggested his contemporary physicians to cure the 'Man' (or Immune System) by using similar symptoms-producing-toxic substances. He failed to provide proofs in support to his proposition except those empirical successes attained by the 'like cure like' process. He failed to explain why symptoms of diseases should not be cured with immunosuppressive medicines because he did not know much about the Immune System which has developed over the next 200 years after his death. Truly, he did his best to explain detrimental effects of using suppressive medication; but, his people were not wise enough understand his explanation. He simply told that diseases are the chronic evolutions of the failures of the 'Man' or 'Vital Power'. It meant that suppression of simple diseases with immunosuppressive medicines will turn into serious diseases which are essentially the results of the immune disorders and deficiency. He guessed this evolution of disease, depending on the long term statistical observations. Indeed, any assumption on the basis of such long-term statistical observation was difficult to prove within a short-spanned lab-test. So, he has been ignored by the scientists along this long period. What Hahnemann said about 200 years ago is now being repeated by Modern Immunologists. Immunologists of the modern era are saying that 'fever' or 'itch' or 'skin diseases' or any disease caused by pathogens should not be cured with immunosuppressive medicines because these medicines do not cure at all, and, instead, they interrupt, blindfold and, thereby, prevent the immune system (or Hahnemann's Man) from working in its own way in response to the pathogens or pathogenic conditions.

When Hahnemann advocated about 'treating the *vital force* (or the *man* or the immune power)', frontiers of Hahnemann's contemporary medical industry got infuriated with obstinate naiveté because of their failure to view the *man* or immune power of the organism. But along the passage of time, scientists' discoveries of biological facts such as immunity, defense ability of the organism, effects of immunosuppressive medicines, etc have forced medical scholars to come to a conclusion on the therapeutic strategy which is closely similar to that of Hahnemann. In the following flowchart, the rationales behind the treatment strategies of Homeopathy and Allopathy are described side by side.

THE SCIENCE OF HOMOEOPATHIC IMMUNOLOGY

```
                    ┌─────────────────────────────────────┐
                    │ A man is suffering from Itch,       │
                    │ Psoriasis, fever or any diseases    │
                    │ caused by microorganisms.           │
                    └─────────────────────────────────────┘
```

Hahnemann's proposition: "Do not treat the diseases. If possible, treat the 'Man' or his 'Vital Power'".

Traditionalists' reaction: "Do not treat the disease! What a sheer idiot Hahnemann is! Remove anything that is disturbing you."

Allopaths' proposition 1: "Remove the <u>symptoms</u>. For example, a. if there is a painful boil on your skin, cut it down. b. If you are getting fever, do something to reduce the temperature, i.e. water therapy, ice therapy, etc. c. If any part of your organ is painful, do something to remove the pain. Use some ointments."

Pre-Pasturian Formula of Treatment. This method of treatment always interferes into the Vital Power's or the Man's response to the pathogens or pathogenic conditions.

Allopaths' proposition 2: "Remove the <u>causes of symptoms</u>. For example, a. if some viruses are the cause of boils or ailments, annihilate the viruses. b. Fever is the result of pyretic emissions from affected cells. So, prevent the Pyrogens from being emitted from the cells in danger. c. Pain is the result of interferonal response of the affected cells. So, prevent the affected cells from producing interferons.

Post-Pasturian Formula of Treatment… Example of Modern Quackery…the quackery continues with the Help of Modern Scientific Discoveries. Evidence-based modern Immunology grows. Physicians learn more accurately about how the 'Vital Force' or 'Man' or 'Immune System' works. So, they begin to use this knowledge to choke (and eventually to destroy) the immune system more accurately.

Postmodern Allopaths' realization: "Symptoms are the responses of the Immune system to the pathogens or pathogenic conditions. So, it is more important to help the Immune System by annihilating the pathogens with antibiotics than to remove symptoms such as fever, itching or boils artificial.

Postmodern Allopaths' realization that "Help the Immune System by annihilating the pathogens, not by disturbing the Immune functions (revealed as symptoms)" is almost similar to the Homoeopathic concept of "Treating the man, not the disease". But if there is no visible pathogen, such traditionalists have failed to answer what should be the process of treating any pathogenic conditions which are not caused by any pathogens.

Hahnemann's proposition: "So! do something which can stimulate or provoke the 'Man' or his 'Vital Power' to take necessary measures against the aggravations".

12

Please take a look at the bottom of the above mentioned flowchart. The left flow shows Hahnemann's proposition to treat the *man* when the *man* falls ill. Such proposition necessarily infers that stimulating or provoking the *man* against the invading threat can help the *man* to get rid of the symptoms of the ailments. On the contrary, the right flow shows the step-by-step changes in the perceptions of the allopaths about how diseases should be cured. Louis Pasteur's discovery of germs as the cause of disease and Metchnikoff's discovery of immune system play two crucial roles in changing the strategies of treatment. First, before Pasteurl's discovery, physicians' sole target was focused on hiding the symptoms by any means such as surgery, bloodletting, scouring, etc. But after the discovery of germs, the physicians aimed at killing the germs and Metchnikoff's discovery of immune system to reach the conclusion that symptoms are the responses of the Immune system to the pathogens or pathogenic conditions. So, it is more important to help the Immune System by annihilating the pathogens with antibiotics than to remove symptoms such as fever, itching or boils artificial. Eventually Alexander Fleming's penicillin helped them in achieving this target, through in chronic cases, the use of antibiotics proved to be quite futile. However, with the increasing knowledge of immune science, scholars explained that antibiotics fail because of the chronic immune-failure to develop effective resistance against the germs. All these immunological conclusions closely resonate what Hahnemann told two centuries ago. Medical scholars took almost two hundred years to understand the role of *vital foirce* or immune system in cure. What do you think how difficult it was for Hahnemann's contemporary scholars to understand Hahnemann's *vital force*?

Another important failure, for which homoeopathy has so far been unsuccessful to garner the acknowledgement of modern science, is Hahnemann and his followers' futile attempt to develop a strong theoretical basis for Homoeopathy. Despite the innumerous successes, they failed to explain how the 'like cures like' concept works and how Homoeopathic medicines work to promote health conditions. We do not know whether they can be excused for this failure; but there is one thing we can say for sure: It was not possible for Hahnemann and his school to explain those two hypotheses without the knowledge of modern immunology. Though Hahnemann attempted to explain it in his own way, his contemporary medical society did not pay heed to him. At places of this book, I described why Hahnemann's contemporary medical scholars avoided his teachings. However, despite their failures in the theoretical field, Homoeopathy has achieved successes in innumerous cases and survived all through these two hundred years.

The efficacy of Homoeopathic medicines is proved statistically. Thousands of cases of patients who have been treated by the homoeopaths around the world will ratify this claim. What is the science that cured all those suffering humanities? Certainly I will explain it. But you (the readers) have to answer my questions first. We want to see if your answers resonate with the Homoeopathic philosophic aspects or the allopathic ones.

Case One: Suppose, a poor neighbor of yours is sick and you, upon being informed, have gone to visit her. The signs of the housewife's sickness are evident everywhere in her house. Everything, the clothes, the utensil, the dining table, the kitchen, etc in the house is in a haphazard condition. How everything had changed after her sickness! She has no near relative to take her to the doctor. What is the best policy to help this sick woman? Will you visit her every day until her death and take care of her? Or will you take her to a good doctor so that she comes round and take care of herself.

Case Two: Suppose you have employed a night guard in order to save your life and wealth from the dacoits and thieves. One night, he started to shout for help. What would you do in such situation? Will you hold him accountable for shouting at dead night and disturbing your sleep? Or will you immediately get up, inquire and take action to help the night guard.

Case Three: Suppose your cherry orchard has been infected by some rats. They are digging up soil from the yard. The orchard is being destroyed. There are piles of soils everywhere. What will you do to save your orchard from the rats? Will you wither all the cherry bushes out so that the rats do not get any cherry to eat and leave the orchard being disappointed of the tantalizing juicy fruits? Or will you simply remove the piles of soil from time to time? Is there any guaranty that the rats will not dig up more? Or will you inquire into the matter and take necessary steps to kill the rats?

In all the three cases,[10] the commoners' answers are obvious. Obviously a man with little bit of common sense will assert that the best strategy to solve the above mentioned problems is to inquire deep and take steps in regard to what is necessary. Obviously all the three cases are intended for the commoners who do not have much knowledge of medical science. Also they are intended for some allopathic Tomboys who would rather keep their eyes closed being driven by rigid antagonism against Homoeopathy. Later I will discuss how and where this antagonism of the allopaths evolves from. Those Tomboys are well equipped with the knowledge, theories, propositions, assumptions and mathematical equations of modern science. Yet they do not understand the obvious truths of Homoeopathic philosophy of Cure. So I am left with no other choice but to put the abovementioned layman's examples to make the truth of Homoeopathic Philosophy more palatable for those

---

[10] These three cases have been an amplification of James Tyler Kent's analogy of the sick man which has been narrated in the Lectures on the Homoeopathic Philosophy

Tomboys' sophisticated mind.

If I say, any commoners' solutions for all the three above-mentioned situations are homoeopathic, will you believe? Let me prove. For the first situation, the most reasonable solution is to treat the 'sick housewife'. Why? It is because if you visit the sick housewife's house from time to time and attempt to keep her house neat and clean instead of taking her to a doctor, all your attempts and efforts are either foolish or shrouded under deceptive motif to win big-hands from others. You deceptively want to show others that you are a gentleman. Let's see what a Homeopath wants to say against the so-called mainstream traditional allopathic medical practice. Suppose,

> You saw a man with a painful, reddish and chronic tumor-like swelling on his wrist. It occurred to the patient for a long time, probably, for years. It is oozing offensively from time to time. Through the hole, the wrist bone is visible. It is obvious that the muscle around the wound is rotting. At first sight, anyone would call it 'possible cancer'.

Here, we will see how the medical professionals respond to the 'possible cancerous swelling'. There are two main approaches to the swelling in regard to the question, "Why the swelling occurs?" and "How the swelling should be cured?" Indeed, the possible answers of these two cardinal questions have been determined by the question "what is disease?" The concept of disease has evolved in different forms in different ages and has influenced the contemporary medical practices as well. Let's see how this medical view of 'disease' has evolved from time to time and how it has compromised with Homoeopathic concept of 'disease'. Though the ancient Chinese and the ancient Egyptian medical practices were derived from some crude philosophical vantages, the rest of the world did not have any strong philosophical concept of 'what disease is' and 'how it should be cured' until the renaissance in Europe during the seventeenth century. The Egyptian and the Chinese Medical philosophies could not satisfy the rational minds of the renaissance scholars. So, a school of renaissance scholars emphasized on the need to delve deep into the role of biological functions of human anatomy in ailment and sufferings. Obviously, there was no clear demarcation between the two concepts, 'disease' and 'suffering' until Luis Pastor's discovery of 'the theory of microorganism'. The following is how the concept of 'disease' changed from time to time after the Renaissance age:

Before Luis Pastor's discovery of 'the theory of microorganism', sufferings and symptoms of a disease themselves were considered as the disease itself. Accordingly, diseases were named according to their symptoms such as fever, cough, choryza, conjunctivitis, tumor, psoriasis and innumerous others which you yourself will find in any medical book at your hand. This deficiency of any clear difference between 'disease' and 'symptoms' misguided the contemporary medical practitioners and provoked them to treat the symptoms only. Their strategy of treating the symptoms was indeed to hide those symptoms at any cost. A good epitome of such quackery was to cut down the tumor or any tumor-like swelling. Such quackery still exists in modern form and appearance in modern medical practice. The same idea, the same philosophy, the same mistake and the same quackery, but with sharper knives and powerful antibiotics in the operation theatre! Surgeons are now more enlightened with specific knowledge of biology, anatomy and medicine. But they will cut one tumor; but they cannot guarantee that another one will not occur. It is because they have removed or cured only the patient's symptom, not his disease. Indeed, they do not have much headache about 'what the disease really is'. Hahnemann vehemently opposed this practice of treating only the symptom. He proposed that treating only the symptoms would not stop its recurring. In order to stop the recurring symptom, the cause (in homoeopathic term, the disease) behind the symptom must be treated. The reasoning behind this homoeopathic concept of 'disease' is quite simple:

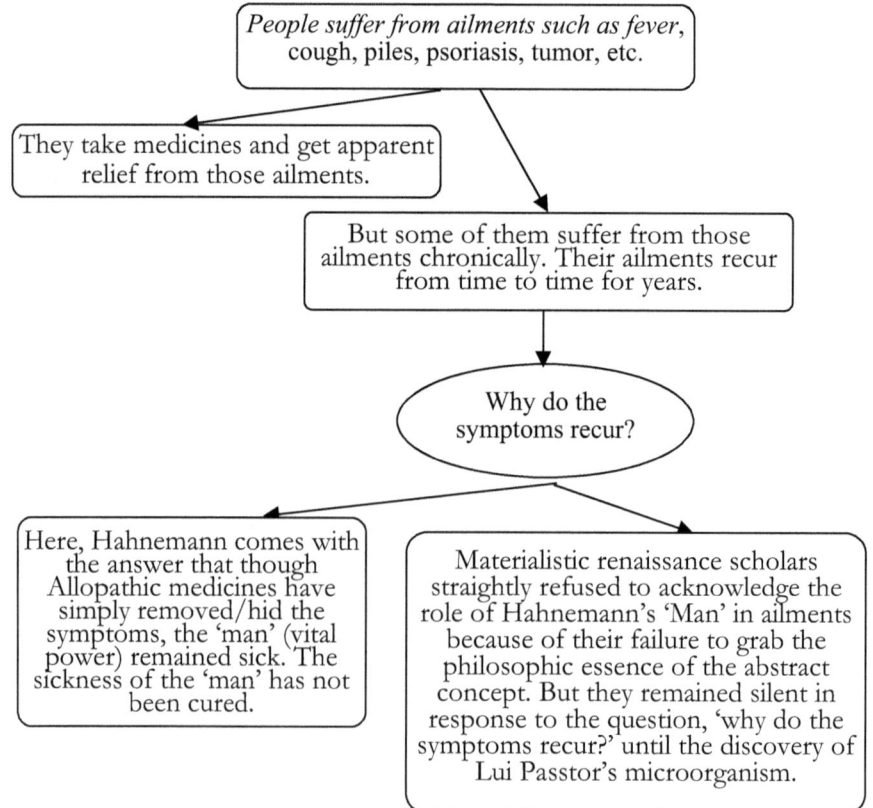

After the discovery of Louis Pasteur's 'microorganism', medical scholars argued that the stronger the organisms are, the longer the course of treatment is. That is, if the pathogenic microorganisms are strong, the symptoms will recur along a long period of time. Here again, the Homoeopathic scholars came up another argument:

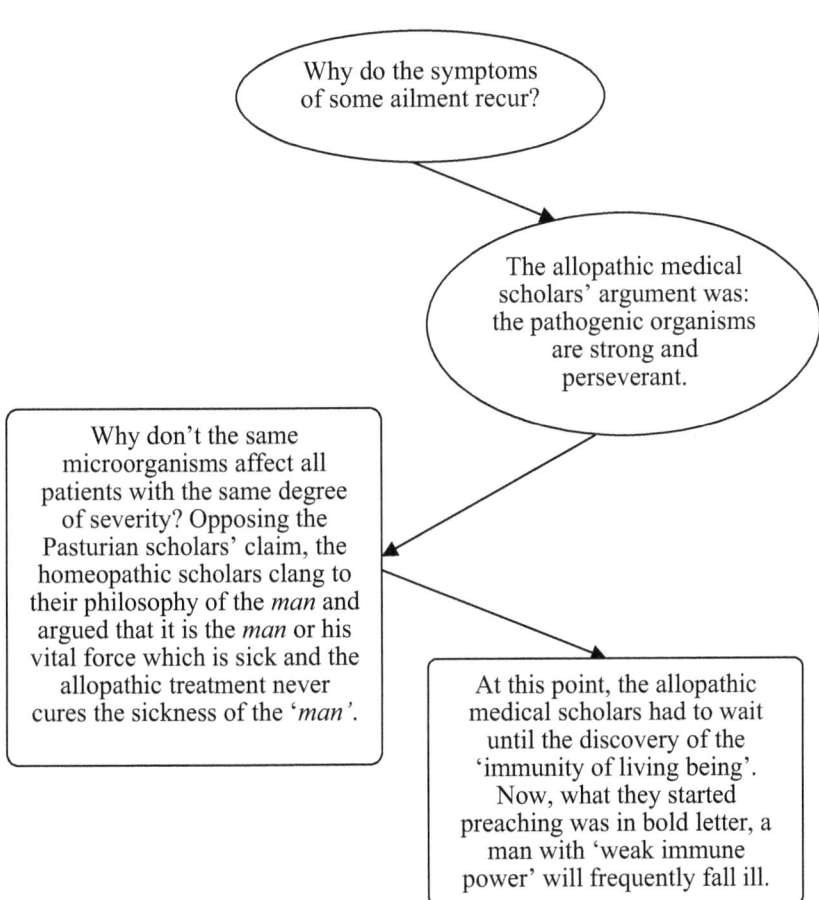

WHOLENESS OF HOMEOPATHIC PHILOSOPHY OF THE *MAN*

Here, please note that what the allopathic scholars identified as the 'immune power' is closely similar to what Hahnemann called 'the man' or the 'vital power'. Yet the Hahnemann's concept is broader, more philosophic and more abstract. Whereas the broadness of the homoeopathic concept of the 'man' covers a wide range of aspects of the *man*'s existence, such as his wellbeing, his ailments, his lifestyle and even how his ailments should be cured, the allopathic concept of 'immune power' is obviously an objective one which never infers what strategy should be taken to cure a patient from ailments. Look at what Hahnemann views the *man's existence*:

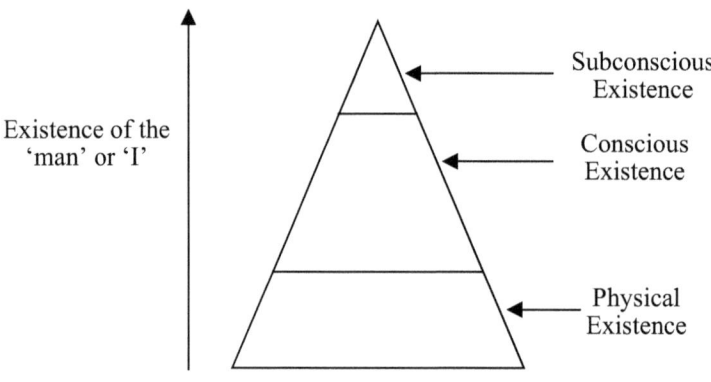

Hahnemann's concept of the 'man' necessarily infers that the 'man's wellbeing' is the totality of the wellbeing of all the three levels of existence i.e. subconscious wellbeing, conscious wellbeing and physical welbeing, as Hahnemann advised that a sincere physician must consider the following: "*the evident physical constitution of the patient (especially in chronic affections), his affective and intellectual character, his activities, his way of life, his habits, his social position, his family relationships, his age, his sexual life, etc.*"[11] Therefore, the 'wellbeing' is the result of the sound performances and wellness of all the three levels of existence. If any or all of the three levels of the existence of the 'man' are sick, the sufferings are visible physically, mentally and existentially. This assertion of homoeopathic 'wellbeing of the man' undeniably says that a patient's sickness does not belong to any single level of the existence of the 'man'. Since all the

---

[11] Samuel Hahneman, *Organon of Medicine*, Para-9

three levels are intertwined with each other, the sickness of one may affect the performance of others resulting into the complication of the visible sufferings. So, this view of the 'man' asserts that the doctor must identify the sickness of the 'man' and treat it accordingly.

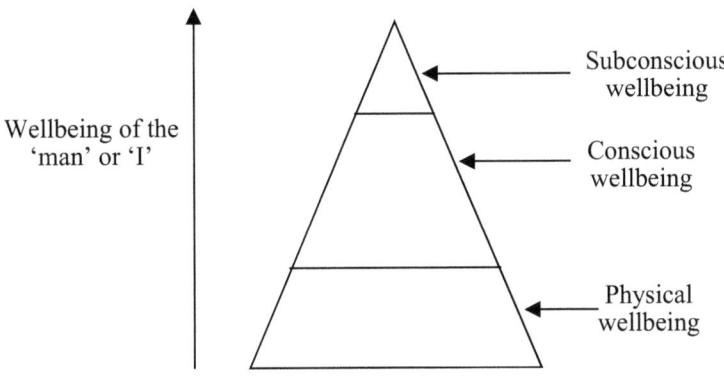

The wholeness of this homoeopathic concept of the 'man' does not permit the homoeopaths to overlook what the 'man's existence' inherits from his ancestors. He must know what is going on in his subconscious mind and how his subconscious existence is endangered and sick. The doctor also should delve deep into the conscious mind to see if there is something disturbing the wellbeing of the 'man'. The interrelation among these three levels are so intertwined with each other that it is an imperative for the homoeopaths to inquire into several issues whatever the ailments (off course, chronic) of the patients are. A homoeopath must look into whether the man or the immune system suffers from any of the followings: a. mental stress and drawback, b. acquired physical drawbacks, c. suppression of immune response, d. failure of immune response, e. injurious effects of lifestyle, f. inherited (genetic) physical drawback, g. accidental physical stress, f. many others

Here, please note that whatever the disease is, if a homoeopath finds that a patient underwent mental grief with the following symptoms of "sighing, sleeplessness, silent tears, easily take offense, etc", he would prescribe Natrum Mur, Ignatia, Pulsatilla, etc with other complementary medicines. Believe it or not, my experience show that the same Natrum Mur cured a whole range of symptoms such as amenorrhea, sleeplessness, sciatica pain, back-pain, psoriasis and many others. If you don't believe, investigate into the efficacy of Natrum Mur and collect data from the homoeopathic doctors and the patients who have been cured by this duo of Natrum Mur and Ignatia. If you find that my claim is factual, then perform researches on the pharmacodynamics and pharmacokinetics of the homoeopathic medicines i.e. Natrum Mur, Ignatia, Pulsatilla, etc. Until you come up with the results of your researches, we have an explanation of why the same medicines work for a number of diseases or symptoms. Look at the following reasoning:

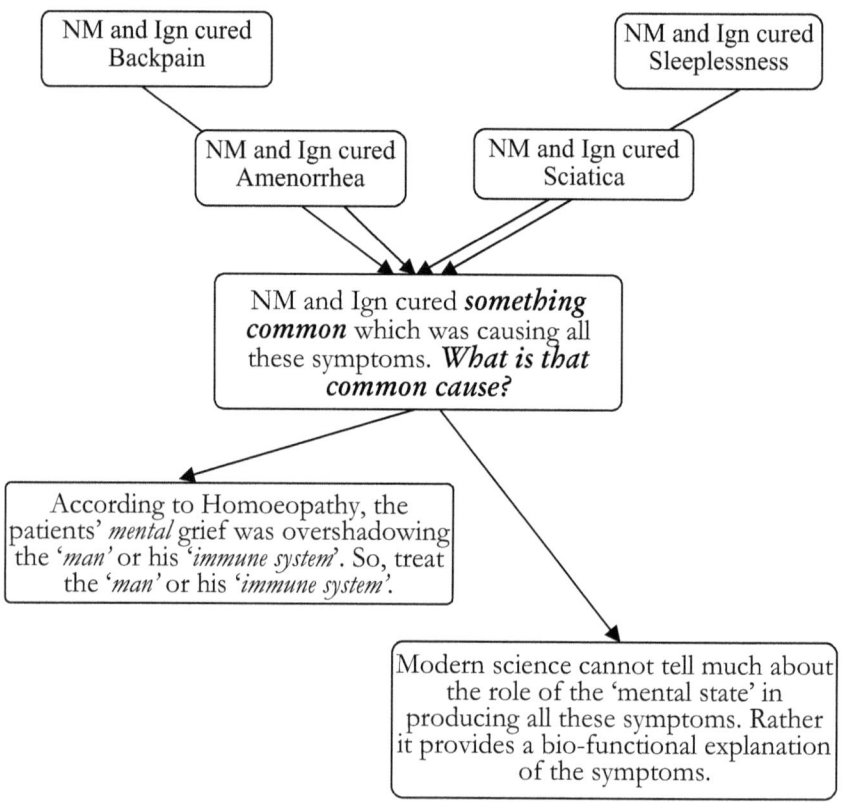

In fact, human biology can provide an individual biofunctional explanation for each of the ailments in the abovementioned diagram. Let's see how medical scholars explain these ailments and their respective treatment strategies:

Most of the medical scholars define amenorrhea mainly as a hormonal disturbance from the hypothalamus, though there are few other anatomical causes such as uterine tumor, pituitary tumors, uterine scars, thyroid problems, etc. So, hormonal medicines along with surgical options are prescribed to correct the problem amenorrhea. Can you find any flaws in these allopathic treatment strategies? Hormonal medication can restart the menstrual period within a very short time. But though some can stop the medication without facing further problems, the problem returns to most of the patients after stopping the medication. The allopathic scholars often like to remain silent to the question why the amenorrhea returns after medication because they know quite well that their hormonal supplies do not cure the disease at all; rather those hormonal supplies temporarily help the organism to continue the menstrual cycle until it takes over the cause which was preventing the production of the hormones. When the organism fails to get the upper hand over the cause, amenorrhea returns immediately after the cessation of the medication. Here we need Hahnemann again. If the allopaths would treat the cause for which the organism fails to produce the necessary hormones for starting the menstrual period, the patient rolled back to a healthy state. Again, an allopathic physician will most probably prescribe, to an insomnia patient, sedatives most of which work by affecting the neurotransmitter gamma-aminobutyric acid (GABA). Indeed, the mechanism of most of the allopathic medicines which either suppress, induce or provide supplement to affect the functions of the organism from without.

Indeed, modern science can provide a biofunctional explanation for each of the diseases (including sleeplessness, sciatica and back-pain) in their pathology books. Such bio-functional explanations necessarily envisage a treatment policy of either suppressing or providing supplements to the bio-functions of each of the diseases with the repetition of age-old faults. On the contrary, Hahnemann's universal policy of treating the *man* requires the physicians to dig up the underlying causes for which the *man* is failing in the specific cases. Even if it is impossible to exhume the underlying cause of the *man's failure*, a homoeopath can reawaken the *man* to address its own problem by terrorizing the *man* with the help of homoeopathic medicines. A deep insight into the cure-pattern (which is shown in the preceding diagram) will compel anybody to ask why and how the same medicines i.e. Natrum Mur and Ignatia in this case can cure diseases of different biofunctional causes. The chemical properties of Natrum Mur and Ignatia do not have the remotest relationship with the hormonal regulation of human body. Even they do not have any relaxation effects on the sciatica nerve. Furthermore you will find that the chemical substances of these two homoeopathic medicines do not have the least effect on the 'neurotransmitter called gamma-aminobutyric acid (GABA)' which is responsible for inducing sleep by slowing down the brain activity. Yet how do they cure all these diseases of different biofunctional basis? How do they cure all the diseases- sleeplessness, amenorrhea, sciatica, etc? If you think allopathically, the pharmacodynamics of these medicines is an endless maze. You must think homeopathically if you want an answer to this question. However, for the time being, you should keep in your head that these two homoeopathic medicines can terrorize the *man* or *immune system* in such a constructive and indicative way that it feels the urgency to spring to action against the functional disturbances. In the abovementioned cases, Natrum Mur and Igantia provoke the immune system (obviously by threatening it) to take initiatives against the threats of Ignatia and Natrum Mur, and, subsequently, against the mental disorders which cause all the above mentioned diseases. Here, please note that though the allopaths use some mental relaxation medications, they are not effective as those homoeopathic medicines because their mechanisms do not have any direct or indirect relations with the organism's *vital force* or immune system.

Whereas, in Homoeopathy, 'mind' is considered an essential part of the 'man' (or the 'immune system') and therefore, of the wellbeing, either mental or physical, of the 'man', for the Allopaths 'mind' is a standalone part, of human being, which plays a very few selective roles in the physical wellbeing of the man. So, an allopath would most probably prescribe different REMEDIES for each of the above mentioned symptoms. Until the discovery of Immune system and the effect of mind's wellbeing on it, prescribing a mind tranquilizer for sciatica pain was utterly confusing for most of the scholars. But now, a good allopath is often found to take mental state into consideration and to prescribe the sedatives for their patients. The medical scholars began to understand most recently what Hahnemann understood almost 250 years ago about the role of mind in the immune system. If a homoeopath asks a patient suffering from Amenorrhea whether she underwent terrible mental grief, any medical scholar of Hahnemann's contemporary era would be drooled to laugh at the choice. But knowledge of modern immunology has changed the situation in Homeopaths' favor.

However, anyone may think that Natrum Mur-Ignatia and the allopathic sedatives are equivalent to each other. But I would desperately say that there is a vast difference between these two types of medicines. Whereas the Homoeopathic medicines are meant to awakening the 'man' and encouraging it to get up and take charge of his decaying household, most of the allopathic medicines are the lullabies (in palliative treatment) which are meant to knock out the 'man' and to keep him in the darkness about what is happening to it. Also, supplementation, another commonly used allopathic treatment strategy, grossly overlook the question what the physicians should do if the organism fails to produce the supplemented materials on its own. Indeed, their advocacy for lifelong medication surprisingly reveals their failure to put faith in the *organism's* ability (immune system) to roll back to its healthy state. Evidences show that such external supplements cause the related organs (where they are produced in) to feel so much pampered that they stop their natural functions of producing the required substances. Gradually, the organs become dead.

Indeed, I made a very much generalized comment on the allopathic medicines. Let me be more specific on what the medicines do and the fallacy behind their use. A general classification of how the medicines work is as following: a. Interfering (killing or inhibiting the growth of) the invading germs, b. destroying the abnormal cells that cause diseases, c. Replenishing the deficient substances (such as hormone and vitamins), d. Change the ways how the cells works, e. Changing the functions of the body to normalize the distress. Depending on the mode of action of the medicines which are currently being used by human societies, the grades of these treatment methods can be determined as following:

a) First Grade Treatment (Homoeopathic): The modes of treatment which can train, develop, strengthen, develop and restore the immune system can be considered as the 'First Grade Treatment'. This mode of treatment does not interfere into or suppress any of the functions of the immune system. Supplementary medication and food-values should help this treatment. Future discoveries about the methods of using immune responses therapeutically will necessarily facilitate the growth of First Grade Medicines (Homoeopathic medicines), while annihilating the others.

b) Second grade treatment (antibiotics and chemotherapies) aims at killing and removing pathogens or pathogenic condition with or without disparaging stress on the immune system. This is not any permanent cure process. Since the Immune System remains the same as before, the symptoms of the diseases may return again and again until the Immune System grows immune tolerance or effective immune defense against those pathogens and pathogenic conditions. If the body fails to grow effective immunity against the sufferings in the long term, the patient needs to depend on the medicine throughout his/her lifetime.

c) Third grade Medicine (suppressive medication) is the utmost deception in the name of treatment. It simply suppresses the immune system, forces it to shut-up and hide the sufferings as long as the medicines remain active. Third Grade medicine will bring temporal relief with real cure by deceiving the Immune system. The long-term treatment with these medicines will bring about tremendous damage to the Immune System and paving the way to serious immunodeficiency and, autoimmune and disordered immune diseases.

d) Fourth Grade treatment process involves removing the affected organs having no real cure. Sometimes, it is the only viable option for a physician.

Let's dissolve each of the allapathic fallacies of using the abovementioned medicines for the regarding diseases. We also endeavor to determine which grade of medicines the allopathic medicines, according to their mode actions, belong to. First we will look deep into how the medicines cure your pain. Even prior to it, we will know what 'pain' is in order to dig up what the allopaths treat under the disguise of science. In this regard, let me remind you of the second case which I mentioned earlier in this article:

> Suppose you have employed a night-guard in order to save your life and wealth from the dacoits and thieves. One night, he started to shout for help. What would you do in such situation? Will you hold him accountable for shouting at dead night and disturbing your sleep?

Certainly, it is the idiocy and severe madness to keep your night-guard's mouth shut when he is supposed to shout for help. The science of Immunology says that 'pain' or 'inflammation' is almost analogous to the night-guard's "shout for help". In an article, "Interactions between the immune and nervous systems in pain", Ke Ren and Ronald Dubner notes,

> Injury to tissue and nerves initiates an inflammatory response that is intended to contain pathogens, clear damaged tissues and promote repair. As one of the five cardinal signs of inflammation, pain (dolor) is initially protective and beneficial to recuperation.[12]

Again look at what the National Health Institute of the USA says: "Pain is a signal in your nervous system that something may be wrong."[13] That is, a part (cell or tissue) of the 'man' (according to the homoeopathic discourse) or the 'immune system' (according to the modern immunology) is suffering and it is shouting for help. It is urging that the immune system or the vital power should take necessary initiatives against the affection. The higher the level of the affection is, the severer the pain (or the more earnest the call for help). Right at this point, an allopath will prescribe "acetaminophen" or "ibuprofen". It means, he mildly scolds your immune system, "shut up". Temporarily, your affected cells stop communicating your brain. After few days, the affected cells begin to shout (pain) again. This time, "acetaminophen" or "ibuprofen" won't work because the threat is severe and complicated. The affected cells need serious attention from you as well as

---

[12] Ke Ren and Ronald Dubner. "Interactions between the immune and nervous systems in pain", NCBI. https://www.ncbi.nlm.nih.gov/pmc/articles/PMC3077564/
[13] Medicineplus. "What is pain?", US National Library of Medicine. https://medlineplus.gov/nondrugpainmanagement.html

your immune system. Again, your doctor will scold him but, this time, with more powerful painkillers such as Percocet, Vicodin, tramadol, Norco, etc. The patient is still suffering from the sickness or the affection; but the patient would never know what is destroying her silently. She as well as her immune system will not take necessary repercussive attempt to check the affection and disease. Are not the painkillers your silent killers? What punishment should be given to those quacks for such deceptive attempt to keep you and your immune system in darkness? Such painkillers are the epitome of quackery in the name of modern science. Please take a look at the following how quackery has evolved with the knowledge of science:

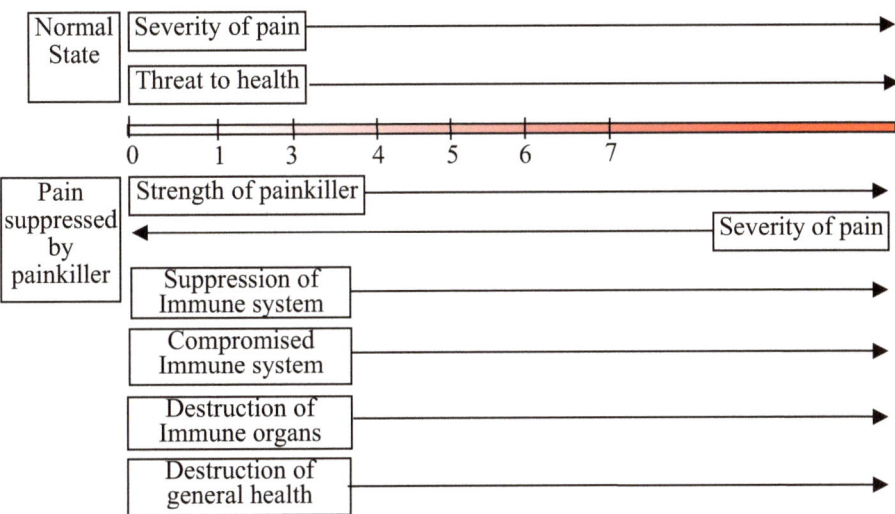

In painful state, the destruction of health is slower than the pain-suppressed state. This pain should not be mitigated through the suppression and compromise of the immune system through painkillers. Instead, the threat which is causing the pain should be addressed. Hahnemann perceived this reality 200 hundred years ago. He earnestly opposed such quackery in the name of treatment. He coined a term "suppression" to refer to such 'deceptive killing' in the name cure. Obviously he was the first to unveil this veil of cure. Now, you will find tones of articles against the side-effects of painkillers. Those authors will tell you that these painkillers will cure your pain, arthritis, sore, inflammation, etc not only at the rate of your hard earned money but also at the rate of the followings:

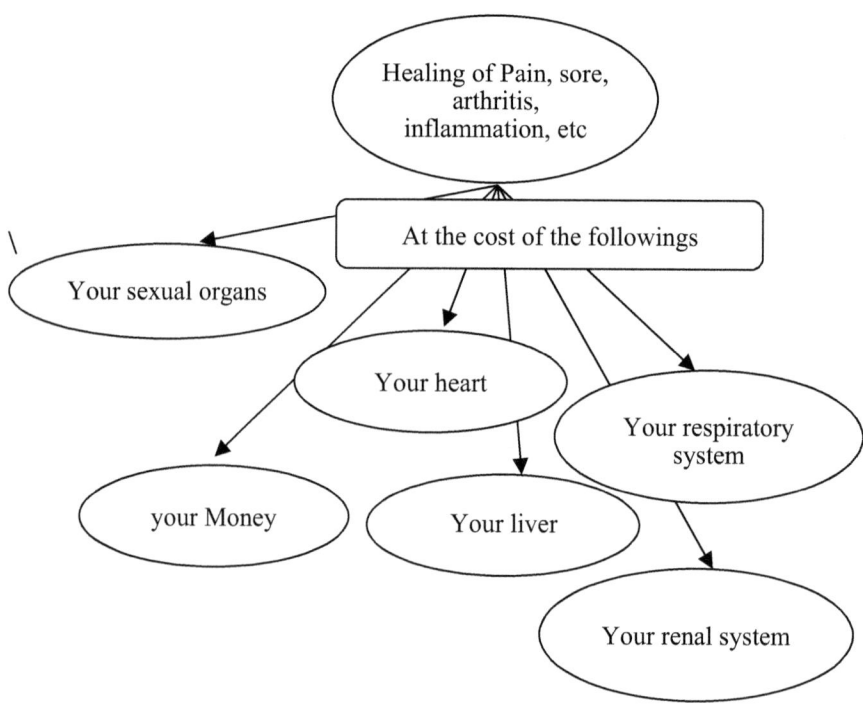

Indeed, these articles will tell you that all the above-mentioned side-effects are the results of the toxicity of the material substances which are used in those so-called medicines. But what they cannot see or simply they do not want to see is the suppression of the 'man' or 'immune system'. It is because if they acknowledge the 'suppression of the man' their so-called medicines will turn into the mostly dreaded piles of toxic substances. In human body, these medicines play a twofold destructive role. First, they themselves are toxic and secondly, they bring about irreversible changes to the immune system (or the *man*) by continually obstructing and suppressing its normal functions. The suppression caused by these medicines is more important than the toxicity of these allopathic medicines. I think, any toxic substance is less harmful than any medicinal substance with the same toxicity along with its suppressive properties. Let's prove it:

Suppose, any toxic substance X (which does not have suppressive power on your immune system) can cause damage to the cells of any organs of your body. Now, your body will necessarily produce antitoxins Y1, Y2, Y3……Yn along with a whole array of other immune responses Z1, Z2, Z3…….Zn

So,
Toxin X ≈ immune responses (Z1+ Z2 + Z3…….Zn) + subsequent antitoxins (Y1+ Y2+ Y3……Yn)

Now, imagine that the toxin X is endowed with the ability of suppressing your immune system. In such case, your immune system will not be able to produce immune responses (Z1+ Z2+ Z3…….Zn) and subsequent antitoxins (Y1+ Y2+ Y3……Yn) against any allopathic toxic medicinal substances. So, it is expected that such immunosuppressive toxic medicines will cause the utmost damage to your health.

Indeed, the ramifications of such immunosuppressive medicines overshadow their toxicity. Hahnemann's 'suppression' is an abstraction of what modern medical science refers to as immunosuppressant. He knew nothing about the immune system; but his concept of the 'man' is even greater and broader than the 'immune system'. So, despite the fact that what he wanted to mean by the term, 'suppression' was observational and empirical, his concept of the man was sufficient enough to forecast the ramifications of the allopathic medicines. He did not know anything about all those terms and concepts of modern immunology. Yet his observations on the clinical data of cures by allopathic medicines helped him to reach a modern conclusion, that is, "suppression" is merely deceptive removal of symptoms without addressing the real diseases and, therefore, it allows the diseases to sit deep rooted within the body of the patient. Later, the frontiers of Homoeopathy developed the concept of 'suppression' more. For convenience, we will consider few of their definitions of suppression. In his book, "Yasgur's Homeopathic Dictionary", Jay Yasgur writes that suppression is "the act of driving a disease deeper inward, against Hering's Law".[14] In the glossary of Samuel Hahnemann's "Organon of the Medical Art", Wenda Brewster O'Reilly explains Hahnemann's concept of "suppression" as "forcible concealment, masking, or forcing under." She further says, "The suppression of symptoms refers to the concealment of perceptible

---

[14] Ann Jerome Croce. "The Thought Behind the Action - Understanding suppression", National Center for Homoeopathy.
https://www.homeopathycenter.org/homeopathy-today/thought-behind-action-understanding-suppression

manifestations of a disease condition without the cure of the disease."[15] Indeed, the homoeopathic concept of 'suppression' reveals three points: 1. leaving the disease unaddressed, 2. forcible concealment of the symptoms, 3. driving the disease deeper inward. Observations of the long-term effects of suppression helped Hahnemann to envisage the three stages (i.e. Psoriatic, Sycotic and syphilitic stages) of the deterioration of the immune system. Indeed, Hahnemann was the first man in human history who successfully handled the concept of immune-deficiency in treatment.

---

[15] Ann Jerome Croce. "The Thought Behind the Action - Understanding suppression"

3
HAHNEMANN'S *MIASM* AND *VITAL FORCE*: EQUIVALENT TO MEDIEVAL MIASMA THEORY AND "VITALISM"?

Those of the critics who dismiss the homoeopathic miasmic interpretation of diseases as a medieval fallacy of the cause of disease must reread the homoeopathic concept of *miasm* and their usages in homoeopathic treatment. It is because the homoeopathic concept of *miasm* does not have the least relation with the obsolete miasma theory which, in the very first place, attempts to explain how infectious diseases spread. Once upon a time, I asked a homoeopath about 'miasm' and his reply was: "Miasms are the causes of diseases and all the human diseases are caused by the three miasms: Psora, Sycosis and Syphilis". I was really appalled by the answer. How, in the world, is it possible that all those diseases (when modern science says that most of the diseases are caused by respective microorganisms such as viruses, bacteria, etc.) are caused by only three miasms? Either the answer of that homoeopath on *miasm* was inept or I was not wise enough not to be misguided by it. I strayed from the science of Homeopathy like many other unfortunates and stayed away for more than 10 years. However, is homoeopathic *miasm* really anything of that obsolete medieval miasma theory? Let see what the prominent homeopaths tell about it. In an article, "Miasms in Classical Homeopathy", David Little tells about "Miasm" as following: "Therefore, in Hahnemannian Homoeopathy the word "miasm" means the effects of microorganisms on the *vital force* including the symptoms that are transmitted to the following generations".[16] As David Little says, Homoeopathic *miasm* refers to "the effects of microorganisms on the *vital force*". In another article "The Thought Behind the Action - Miasms: Psora, Syphilis, Sycosis", Ann

---

[16] David Little. "Miasms in Classical Miasms in Classical Homeopathy", Homoeo Academe Journal.
https://sites.google.com/a/homoeoacademe.com/journal1/miasms-in-classical-homoeopathy-part-i-david-little

Jerome Croce defines *miasm* as following:

> The story of miasms begins with Samuel Hahnemann himself……Hahnemann found that chronic diseases arise from a <u>deep inner susceptibility</u> that he called miasm. External causes of disease, he observed, can bear fruit only in the fertile ground of a miasmatic foundation, which passes by various means from person to person and creates the predisposition to particular kinds of disease states.[17]

The *miasm* as a 'deep inner susceptibility' is far more different from the medieval concept of *miasm* as the causes of all diseases. The homoeopathic *miasm* as a 'deep inner susceptibility' is a quite eloquent prediction of the 'man' (or 'vital power' or 'immunity'). Hahnemann redefined 'miasm' simply to explain why some patients suffer from some symptoms chronically. Please take a note here. For Hahnemann, it was a challenge to define why some patients suffer from particular symptoms for a long time. He was an empiricist as well as a rationalist. He observed the chronic cases of the patients' illness throughout his career as a physician. He needed to induce conclusions from his observations and to theorize those conclusions as well. In this regard, he had to rely heavily on the existing medical philosophy of '*Vitalism*' which is now considered as an obsolete medical philosophy. But we have a question here: How did Homeopathy survive all those years after its discovery until now depending on an invalid theory? Friedrich Wohler proved Vital Theory invalid by synthesizing urea from nonorganic compounds in the late 1820s.[18] Wohler's synthesis invalidated the principles of Vital Theory. But does it mean that *Vital Theory* has nothing to do with the mysteries of biological science? Indeed, *Vitalism* as a medical philosophy emerged to provide plausible explanations of the realities of biology. When any philosophical concept attempts to explain realities, it only provides abstraction. It is because philosophical envisions, in most cases, precede scientifically proved theories. *Vitalism* as a philosophy inspired Jöns Jacob Berzelius to setting down the vital principles: 1. "Organic compounds cannot be made in the laboratory from inorganic compounds", 2. "Synthesis of organic compounds requires a *vital force*" and 3. "Only living organisms contain *vital force*"[19]. These principles of *Vitalism* which were falsified by Wohler were merely three conclusions drawn by Jacob Berzelius in an attempt to answer the questions why and how the living entities are different from non-living entities.

---

[17] Ann Jerome Croce. "The Thought Behind the Action - Miasms: Psora, Syphilis, Sycosis". National Center for Homoeopathy.
https://www.homeopathycenter.org/homeopathy-today/thought-behind-action-miasms-psora-syphilis-sycosis
[18] Wikipedia. "Vitalism". https://en.wikipedia.org/wiki/Vitalism
[19] Laura Foist. "*Vital force* Theory". Study. https://study.com/academy/lesson/vital-force-theory-definition-principals.html

VITALISM: A LIVING BODY IS EQUAL TO A CORPSE?

Medieval *Vitalism* is nothing of Homoeopathy but is it that useless? We need to look at how *Vitalism* explains the complex difference between the living and the non-living: "living organisms are fundamentally different from non-living entities because they contain some non-physical element or are governed by different principles than are inanimate things".[20] Though the scientists are reluctant to pay *Vitalism* its due respect, it, indeed, can be assessed as a biological assumption of the age-old question of how life is different from death. The inspiration of *Vitalism* is as following. We know that there is a definite difference between a living entity and a non-living entity. The two can never be equal to each other. So, the following is true:

$$A \text{ living entity} \approx a \text{ non-living entity}$$
$$\text{Or, } A \text{ living entity} = a \text{ non-living entity} + x$$
$$\text{Or, } A \text{ living body} = a \text{ non-living body} + x$$

Here, X is what is missing from the non-living entity. Different branches of knowledge define 'X' from different point of views. Obviously this X has a number of derivatives, X1, X2, X3, X4……Xn. So, the following is true:

$$A \text{ living Entity} = a \text{ non-living Entity} + X1 + X2 + X3 + \ldots\ldots + Xn.$$

Where,
X1 = something that says 'I' and that differentiates its 'self' from others.
X2 = something that becomes happy and feels pain at times.
X3 = Functions of the non-living entities to ensure happiness for X1
X4 = Environments for smooth functioning of the functions or X3
Xn = many other undiscovered possibilities and traits of X

X is indeed the variable of which the meaning and attributes have changed from time to time. For the psychiatrists, it is *mind*; for religions, it is the soul; for the biologists, it is *biological functions*. For the mechanists, X in nothing but the systematic activeness of the non-living entity. So, does it mean that X is equal to 0? Can we believe what Mechanistic view of life infers as following?

$$A \text{ living body} = a \text{ non-living body}$$
$$\text{Or, a living man} = a \text{ dead man}$$

Isn't it confusing that we have to believe that a living man is equal to a

---

[20] BECHTEL, WILLIAM and ROBERT C. RICHARDSON. "Vitalism". In E. Craig (Ed.), Routledge Encyclopedia of Philosophy. London: Routledge.
http://mechanism.ucsd.edu/teaching/philbio/vitalism.htm

corpse? Science has ruled out the existence of *soul* because it has some limitations to speak what it cannot argue for, whereas a philosopher enjoys the freedom of imagining the reality which is beyond the perception of the plain eyes. So, the X is, indeed, a philosophical factor which differentiates between a living body and a non-living body. For the Vitalists, it was "some non-physical element" or "different principles" that make the living being different from the non-living. Can we consider the "non-physical element or different principles" analogous to the factor X? Indeed both "different principles" and factor X are the abstraction of the unknown differences between the living and the non-living. Any possible principles of the living beings will be guessed and hypothesized; they will be tested as well; most of them will be falsified whereas few of them will pass the tests of scientific methodologies. The followings are examples of the falsified propositions of *Vitalism*:

Aristotelian concept of abiogenesis: Aristotle's abiogenesis was essentially an attempt to explain one of the unknown aspects of X, that is, if X or *life* can be (or spontaneously is) puffed into any non-living entity overnight. Pasteur's experiments falsified this notion of abiogenesis.

a. Pasteur's experiments established another feature of the X that "*Omne vivum ex vivo*" ("Life only comes from life"). Please note the irony here. Pasteur's experiment debunked one aspect of *Vitalism* whereas establishing another. He established that X is not the result of *Vital force* but of another X.
b. Scientists learnt more about the features of X. They postulated that the simplest forms of Life (that is X) evolved from nonorganic primordial elements. This modern concept of abiogenesis claims, defying the concept of *Vital force*, that life can evolve from non-organic elements. Indeed this view about the evolution of life negates 'life' or X itself because it claims that life (or X/*Vital force*) is nothing but the autonomous functions of entities which are constituted of matters.
c. Another hypothesis about the attributes of the X that "Organic compounds cannot be made in the laboratory from inorganic compounds" was falsified by Wohler's experiments.

If X is the distinction between life and death, *Vitalism* is simply the attempt to explain what the X is. So, *Vitalism* was never an established scientific theory; rather it was an attempt to fill the void of any established scientific theory about living being in the 18th century. However, for Hahnemann, this X was 'vital power'. Hahnemann's concept of 'vital power' is quite different from his contemporary vitalist concept of 'vital power' (or 'force' or Aristotelian Pneuma/vital heat). Medieval concept of 'vital power' (or Vitalism) was put forth to explain the difference between the living entity and the non-living entity, Hahnemann's concept of vital power came as an explanation of how a living entity defends itself from pathogenic agents. Most of his concepts were made from his experiences through inductive reasoning as he said, "Homeopathy lays only over my experience. Do imitate me, but do it well and you shall see at each step the confirmation of my statements."[21] Go through Hahnemann's *Organon of Medicine* you will find that the whole book is laden with statements which show that his concept of *Vital force* is a unique concept in the medical history. In the first half of the 18th century, he began to speak of a mysterious force or power which is:

> In the state of health the spirit-like *vital force* (dynamis) animating the material human organism reigns in supreme sovereignty. It maintaining the sensations and activities of all the parts of the living organism in a harmony that obliges wonderment. The reasoning spirit who inhabits the organism can thus freely use this healthy living instrument to reach the lofty goal of human existence.[22]

HAHNEMANN'S SPIRIT *LIKE VITAL FORCE* AND MODERN IMMUNOLOGY

Imagine, a man of the 18th century who knew nothing about Pasteur's germ theory and Metchnikoff's immune experiment was speaking of a "*spirit-like vital force*" which reigns the "material human organism" in supreme sovereignty. Why did he call it 'spirit-like'? It is because he felt that this *vital force* has its own spirit which has have the power of "reasoning" and continues to function until the death of the man in order for ensuring "the sensations and activities of all the parts of the living organism in a harmony"[23]. This "reasoning spirit" inhabits within our body but we are not much aware of it. It plays an important role in the sensory system of the body and "maintains its vital functions". Furthermore, it animates the material body to defend itself from the "forces of the outer material world". In bold line, it is the defense system of the living organism. So, "without the *vital force* the body dies; and then, delivered exclusively to the forces of the outer material world, it decomposes, reverting to its chemical constituents"[24] He also said that his *vital force* is self-sustaining, as he says in Aphorism 11: "When man falls ill it is at first only this self-sustaining spirit-like *vital force* (vital principle) everywhere present in the organism which is untuned by the *dynamic influence* of the hostile disease-agent".[25] Does he not refer by the phrase "*self-sustaining spirit-like vital force*" to the self-sustaining immune system of human body? Hahnemann's *vital force* is fighter, warrior and strategist. Its every step against its enemies is highly

---

[21] Samuel Hahnemann. "Hahnemann Quotes", http://homeopatia.bvs.br/en/vhl/know-more-about-homeopathy/hahnemann-quotes/
[22] Samuel Hahneman, Organon of Medicine, Para-9
[23] Samuel Hahneman, Organon of Medicine, Para-9
[24] Samuel Hahneman, Organon of Medicine, Para-9
[25] Samuel Hahneman, Organon of Medicine, Para-11

calculative as the modern immune system. It tries heart and soul to thwart threats and overcome its enemies. But sometimes it fails and needs physicians' help. Are not all these features reminiscent of modern immune system. Read the lines from Aphorism 29 and specially note the underlined part:

> Natural diseases (of psoric, syphilitic, and sycotic nature) though weaken than artificial ones have a longer action, nearly always as long as life itself, and <u>cannot be overcome and extinguished by the *vital force* without the help of a therapeutic agent.</u>[26]

No other man in human history told about the '*vital force*' in the way this man spoke. Hahnemann's concepts about the '*vital force*' were confusing to the people who knew nothing about the complex immune system of the body. It was even more confusing when he claimed that disease as what the people of his time perceived is a "state of being of the organism dynamically untuned by a disturbed *vital force*".[27] He further claimed that disease is caused by the *vital force*, as he said, "It is only this *vital force* thus untuned which brings about in the organism the disagreeable sensations and abnormal functions that we call disease."[28] Another such apparently confusing statement about disease is: "It is only the pathologically untuned *vital force* that causes diseases."[29] It was the most confusing statement which drove most of the scholars of his era into bewilderment. This gentleman further added fuel to their bewilderment by severely criticizing the traditional medical practices. Being angered, they threw him out of his country, Germany. Suppose you are a well-educated immunologist who has been sent to Hahnemann's era by travelling by a time-machine and your duty is to teach the people of Hahnemann's society the immune system and its role in disease. Provided that, you will not use the term, *immune system*; you must use the term *vital force* instead. You would use the language (to teach them) what Hahnemann had already done. This is my challenge to the whole non-homoeopathic medical industry to prove wrong the following statement that Hahnemann's *vital force* was the first ever medical concept which is closer than all other preceding medical concepts to the abstraction of modern concept of *immune system*. If you disagree with me, please do some homework and prove me wrong. Here, I want to mention Dr. Stephen Decker's definition of what he thinks as Hahnemann's definition of disease:

> For Hahnemann, disease is a dynamic or supersensible phenomenon that resides above the physical body in what is commonly referred to as the

---

[26] Samuel Hahneman, Organon of Medicine, Para-29
[27] Samuel Hahneman, Organon of Medicine, Para-8
[28] Samuel Hahneman, Organon of Medicine, Para-11
[29] Samuel Hahneman, Organon of Medicine, Para-11

astral body of man, that part of the dynamic man that involves the emotions and desire, what he called a "dynamic affection."[30]

I want to make objection to the use of the terms, "phenomenon that resides above the physical body" and "the astral body of man". Where on earth did he get the references from Hahnemann's writings which attest that the two phrases have anything to do with the homoeopathic medical science? In this book, I quoted so many lines from the *Organon Of Medicine* which clearly show Hahnemann's definition of *disease* is far away from Stephen Decker's perception of supersensible disease "that resides above the physical body in what is commonly referred to as the astral body of man, that part of the dynamic man that involves the emotions and desire". Decker's definition is completely a bogus boo which glaringly exhumes his incapability to understand the immunological feature of Hahnemann's *disease*. I have another objection to the same author's explanation of the disease process. He says, "A disturbance of our natural, god-given desire function then deranges the functioning of the organism and eventually leads to physical symptoms, the famous hierarchy of altered feelings, functions and sensations".[31] I do not know how it is possible to reach such conclusion. This statement of Decker is partially true because the 'disorders and derangements of mind' is one of many factors which detrimentally affect Hahnemann's *vital force*.

So, Hahnemann's *vital force* is quite scientific and what he meant by it is essentially the modern immune system. Therefore, how is it possible that he will consider three miasms as the roots of diseases? Look how a popular website like Wikipedia is spreading rumors about Hahnemann. It says, "Hahnemann believed the underlying causes of disease were phenomena that he termed *miasms*, and that homeopathic preparations addressed these".[32] It further says, "Hahnemann's hypotheses for the direct or remote cause of all chronic diseases (miasms) originally presented only three, psora (the itch)…[which is] supposed to be derived from suppressed scabies".[33] What an irony! Hahnemann's greatest fear was that people will not understand his concepts and therefore his discovery will remain unused. The following is how he expressed his fear:

> But in communicating to the world this great discovery, I am sorry that I must doubt whether my contemporaries will realize the consistency of these teachings of mine…rather leave them untried and unimitated, and therefore unused.[34]

---

[30] Steven Decker, Patty Smith and Rudi Varspoor. "The Dynamic Nature of Disease", Chronic Disease in Dr. Hahnemann's Medical System. Page 17
[31] Stephen Decker et al. "The Dynamic Nature of Disease",
[32] Wikipedia. "Homoeopathy", https://en.wikipedia.org/wiki/Homeopathy
[33] Wikipedia. "Homoeopathy", https://en.wikipedia.org/wiki/Homeopathy
[34] Hahnemann, Chronic Diseases and Their Cure, translation by S.R. Decker,

Truly, he was far more ahead of his contemporary society. I showed earlier how it was difficult for him to convince his people on the idea of *vital force*. Indeed, it is more difficult for Hahnemann's contemporary scholars to perceive *Vital force* than for people in the 21st century. Indeed, Hahnemann's homoeopathy was, indeed, the premature child of modern science. If Hahnemann had knowledge of modern immunology, he could communicate his concept more conveniently. He brought forth the concept of *miasm* to explain why diseases relapse chronically and how to treat them.

CONTROVERSIES ABOUT HAHNEMANN'S *MIASM*: THE CAUSE OF DISEASE?

Whereas Hahnemann's *vital force* was itself a challenge to his contemporary scholars, his *miasm* was, indeed, a mortal blow to their confusion about the challenge. The reaction of Hahnemann's contemporary society to the *miasm theory* was obvious. Dr. Richard Haehl says, "One of the keenest students of this new theory declared in 1836 that he had encountered not one homeopath that agreed with it".[35] Even during these days homoeopaths themselves, let alone the allopaths, are divided in embracing Hahnemann's *miasm theory*. There are some "allopathically-trained homeopaths criticizing Hahnemann's disease classification based on current materially-based and derived disease distinctions, implying that Hahnemann's insights are out of date, crude and can be set aside in the light of modern medical science".[36] However, there are others who will acknowledge and utilize *miasm* successfully in their treatment, but will never make any attempt to explain why it is scientific. The following is how Mohit Mathur tells about *miasm*:

> The concept of *miasm* is one of the most controversial aspects of homeopathy. Their evolution, exact nature and how Hahnemann came to consider them the fundamental cause of both acute and chronic disease are areas where opinions of the homeopaths are divided.[37]

Where does the controversy about *miasm* arise from? Why are the homeopaths around the world divided on this issue? If you go through Hahnemann's *Chronic Disease*, you will note that the concept of *miasm* eludes the readers on several points. First, it is the term *miasm* itself which will allure you to align it with the medieval *Miasma Theory*. Secondly, *miasm* seems to be

---

electronic version
[35] Haehl, Richard, Samuel Hahnemann, His Life and Work, Vol II, p. 148.
[36] Steven Decker, Patty Smith and Rudi Varspoor. "The Dynamic Nature of Disease", Chronic Disease in Dr. Hahnemann's Medical System. P19
[37] Mohit Mathur. "The concept of miasm—evolution and present day perspective", Homeopathy (2009) 98, 177–180

an external force which causes diseases in human body. Thirdly, few traits of Hahnemann's *miasm* have been theorized in ways which are outdated by modern science. Hahnemann's theoretical explanation of *miasm* is partly medieval and mostly scientific though premature. For some mysterious reason, Hahnemann did not use any unique term to explain his concept of *miasm* as well as *vital power*. But a deep exploration of the concept will necessarily force you to feel that the medieval *miasm* and Hahnemann's *miasm* are completely different from each other and the second one is quite antagonistic to the first one. Any medieval connotation of the term *miasm* refers to any external (material or organic) disease producing force which is a putrescent, corrupt, deplete and evil external force like vaporous exhalation which inflicts diseases to body. But Hahnemann's *miasm* is more of a biological deficiency which is mostly genetic and internal. So, those who consider *miasm* as an external disease-causing force are grossly wrong in evaluating Hahnemann's *concept of disease*. Many lines from the *Organon* show that Hahnemann did not have any headache about any external disease producing material or organic agents. Go through the *Chronic Disease*, you will find that Hahnemann marked *Psora* as the most important of three *Miasms*. When you will try to perceive what Hahnemann meant by the term *Psora*, you will see that you are being continually allured to consider the terms, arch malady, itch mites, scabies, etc as the materialistic counterparts of *Psora*. Dr. Steven Decker et al points out the danger of such tendency.

In their book, *Chronic Disease in Dr. Hahnemann's Medical System*, Steven Decker et al says, "the terms that Hahnemann uses for disease, while they may bear a resemblance to existing disease names, are not to be reduced to their material counterparts, or even judged thereby".[38] Indeed, Dr Steven Decker's perception of the abstraction of *miasm* is praiseworthy. But at the same time, I will hold him accountable for not going beyond the literal meaning of Hahnemann's theorization of *disease and miasm,* and not attempting to put forth a scientific explanation of the practical usage of the homoeopathic *disease and miasm* in treatment. The homoeopaths' failure to go beyond the surface meaning of Hahnemann's nosology can be exemplified by Stephen Decker's perception of Hahnemann's definition of *disease*. In the following lines, Decker has tried to explain what, according to Hahneman, causes *disease*:

> A disturbance of our natural, god-given desire function then deranges the functioning of the organism and eventually leads to physical symptoms, the famous hierarchy of altered "feelings, functions and sensations" used in homoeopathic case-taking.[39]

---

[38] Steven Decker, Patty Smith and Rudi Varspoor. "The Dynamic Nature of Disease", Chronic Disease in Dr. Hahnemann's Medical System. P18

[39] Steven Decker, Patty Smith and Rudi Varspoor. "The Dynamic Nature of Disease", Chronic Disease in Dr. Hahnemann's Medical System. P17

This psychophysical interpretation of *disease* of Stephen Decker is not completely compatible with the whole medical system of Hahnemann. Certainly *mind* plays a very important as the cause of *disease* and in the healthy functions of *vital force*. In Hahnemann's medical system, *mind* is one of many factors (I described the factors) which directly or indirectly affect the sound functioning of the *vital force*. But it is not the sole cause of *disease* as Decker claimed. Indeed, "disturbance of our natural, god-given desire function" cannot be the sole cause of Hahnemann's *disease*. Yet if it is considered so, why would Hahnemann say that *disease* is produced by the *vital force* in Aphorism 11? Read the following part from Aphorism 11: "*It is only this vital force thus untuned which brings about in the organism the disagreeable sensations and abnormal functions that we call disease.*"[40] Are *mind* and *vital force* synonymous to each other for Hahnemann? No! they are not synonymous at all.

I do not know how Decker et al came to such conclusion that "a disturbance of our natural, god-given desire function then deranges the functioning of the organism". I am sorry that I failed to trace the true source of such an important claim of Decker et al about the Hahnemannian *disease*. Even though Hahnemann might have mentioned it in one of his books, I am quite sure he did so to explain the effect of mind on the functioning of *vital force* and its role as one of the causes of *disease*. Decker's psychophysical interpretation of *disease* is misleading because it misguides the readers in grabbing the true essences of *miasm*. A careful reading of Hahnemann's *Chronic Disease* and *Organon of Medicine* will necessarily divulge that Hahnemann used the concepts such as miasm, *disease-agent*, Contagion, disease, *vital force*, etc distinctively. Hahnemann was not oblivious to the presence of any external pathogenic agents; he termed it as *disease-agent* (which also connotes the essence of modern 'germ'). He was quite aware of that the *vital force* may be threatened by *disease-agent*. He called it as *contagion*. But he was more concerned with the *unturned state* of *vital force* than with the *disease-agent*. The following lines from the *Chronic Disease* partly reveal the sequence among these terms:

> From the progress of all these miasmatic diseases we may plainly see that, after the contagion from without, the malady connected with it in the interiors of the whole man must first be developed; i.e, the whole interior man must first have become thoroughly sick of smallpox, measles or scarlet fever, before these various eruptions can appear on the skin.[41]

Now, we will draw the sequence in a flow chart:

---

[40] Hahnemann, *Organon of Medicine*. Aphorism 11
[41] Hahnemann, *Chronic Disease*. P. 34

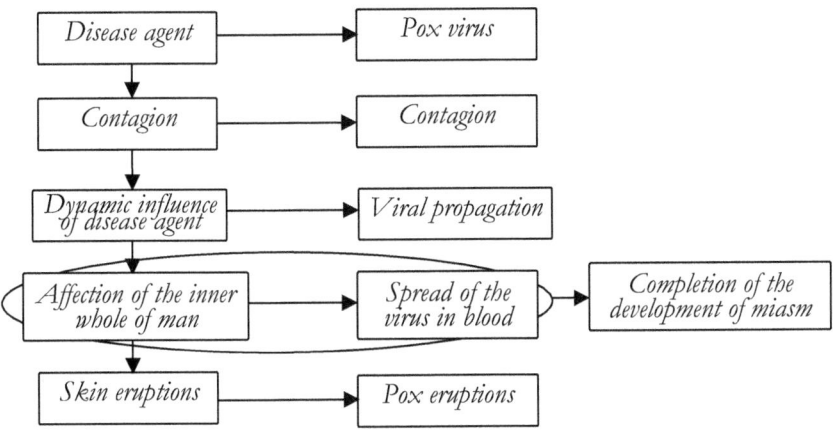

My attempt to keep *disease-agent* at the beginning step of the process of the development of *miasm* is quite justified because the untuned state of *vital force* begins with the "*dynamic influence* of the hostile *disease-agent*".[42] According Hahnemann, the development of the *miasm* becomes complete in the fourth stage when "the whole interior man must first have become thoroughly sick". So, it is clear that *miasm* is caused by the invasion of miasmatic disease and suppressive medication. Here, I do not know how some scholars claim that disease is caused by *miasm*. It is somewhat like claiming that "all those trees i.e. banana tree, banyan tree, jackfruit tree, coconut tree, apple tree, eucalyptus tree, amla plant, etc can be grown from a single seed of mango." Is it possible to grow different trees from a single seed? Did Hahnemann actually claim so? Indeed, such claims have played a great role in making Hahnemann's *miasm* controversial and scientifically implausible. The claim that the same *miasm* i.e. *Psora* as a disease-agent like the germ of any specific disease causes all the psoric diseases such as smallpox, cowpox, measles, psoriasis, ringworm and tons of other skin diseases is scientifically impossible. But *miasm*, for say, *psora* as the immune-deficiency or state of sickness of the *vital force*, makes the organism prone to be affected by all of the psoric diseases. It is something like claiming that "all those trees i.e. banana tree, banyan tree, jackfruit tree, coconut tree, apple tree, eucalyptus tree, amla plant, etc can be grown on this soil."

Hahnemann clearly identified the stage at which the miasmatic deficiency of the *vital force* grows. He notes that it is the fourth stage in which the *vital force* (the inner whole of man) becomes thoroughly sick of the disease and begins to show eruptions on skin, as he says, "thirdly, the breaking out of the

---

[42] Hahnemann, *Organon of Medicine*. Aphorism 11

external ailment, whereby nature externally demonstrates the completion of the internal development of the miasmatic malady throughout the whole organism"[43]. Please note the use of the word 'miasmatic' in the phrase 'the completion of the internal development of the miasmatic malady'. It is remarkable that whenever he used the term 'miasmatic', he did so to refer to something which internally corrupts and defeats the *vital force*.

For Hahnemann, the *disease* is the *untuneness* of *vital force* itself (which is spoken of by the *vital force* in the forms of symptoms). Sound *vital force* can fight of the acute infection within a short duration on its own. In answer to the question why (chronic) disease persists for a long time, Hahnemann guessed that the *vital force* sometimes becomes so much subdued and suppressed by wrong medication, unhealthy practice and lifestyle, detrimental mental health, etc that it can never get the upper hand over the existing *untuneness*. So, the suffering symptoms perpetuate for a long time. Look the question which inspired Hahnemann to conjure up the concept of *miasm*:

> Why, then, cannot this *vital force*, efficiently affected through Homoeopathic medicine, produce any true and lasting recovery in these chronic maladies...? What is there to prevent this?

Hahnemann's reasoning was simple and brilliant. In acute cases, the *vital force* with the help of homoeopathic medicines so effectively fights off the maladies. What prevent the *vital force* from doing so in case of chronic maladies? Since he had little headache for the external *disease-agent*, his prime concern was focused on anything which mutilates the ability of the *vital force*. Hahnemann guessed that it which prevents the *vital force* from fighting off the chronic maladies is more of a type of weakness or subdued state of the *vital force* than of any individual entity. He started using the term, *miasm* in an attempt to define the stages of the deterioration of the untuneness. Many lines from the *Chronic Disease* can be quoted to show that *miasm* itself is neither the disease nor the cause of disease. Rather it is something like the corruption of the whole interior, as Hahnemann wanted to provide an explanation of how *miasm* takes place in human body:

> From the progress of all these miasmatic diseases we may plainly see...the malady connected with it in the interiors of the whole man must first be developed; i.e, the <u>whole interior man</u> must first have become thoroughly sick....[44]

In these lines he shows how miasms are the corruption of the *whole interior of man*. If Hahnemann considered *miasm* as a separate pathogenic entity (like

---

[43] Hahnemann, *Chronic Disease*. P. 32
[44] Hahnemann, *Chronic Disease*. P. 34

germs) causing disease, would he claim that *miasm* is ultimately the result of suppressing the *vital force?* He claimed that *miasmic disease* occurs due to the suppression of the *vital force* with suppressive medications. For him, *miasm* is something internal as he says, "Gradually I discovered more effective means against this original malady…Psora; i. e. , against the internal itch disease with or without its attendant eruption on the skin"[45] The phrase, "*Psora*…the internal itch disease with or without its attendant eruption on the skin" is very much remarkable for the careful selection of words. It means that *Psora* is essentially internal disease. As it is internal, it is not necessary that it will have skin eruptions. However, since *disease* is the *untuned state* of the *vital force*, *Psora* is a particular state of the *untuneness* or disorders of the *vital force*. In the *Psora* stage, the *vital force* loses its ability to fight off the *disease-agent*s or germs through vesicular eruptions and to develop further defense strategy against future infection. This failure of the *vital force* compels the organism to succumb to further threats and gradually takes it to other miasmic stages.

Indeed, Hahnemann's *miasm* has so long been misinterpreted by most scholars who took it for the cause of diseases. If *miasm* is taken in its true essence, that is, as stages of inner immune deficiencies (as Hahnemann wanted to convey), *miasm* is mostly scientific and quite compatible with the discoveries of modern biology. What Hahnemann told about *miasm* and *chronic disease* is essentially the result of his careful observation and research. In most cases, Hahnemann's observations about the biology of human body can be ratified with the theories and discoveries of modern science, though he suffered from the lack of vocabulary tremendously. In an explanation of how *miasm* develops, Hahnemann needed to delve deep into how the *vital force*s (or the immune system) gradually succumb to *miasmatic disease*. Certainly, he needed to classify some diseases as *miasmatic* because these diseases could easily corrupt the *vital force*. So when he used the phrase, 'the miasma of itch', this 'miasma' needs not be considered as the *medieval miasma*. Though he chose to use the same medieval term, he successfully redefined it to fit it into his observations. Furthermore, the fact whether the term 'miasma' connotes medieval essence of disease-agent or disease-carrier or disease-transmitter or not, is of less importance than how the miasmatic disease. It is because, in order for explaining his unprecedented therapeutics, Hahnemann had not only to reconstitute the medieval concept of *vital force* but also to explain how its perpetual *untuneness* grows while fighting with *miasmatic diseases*. It was more important for him to discover why the *vital force* perpetually fails to clear off the *miasmatic disease* and how this failure of the *vital force* pushes the organism towards further deterioration than to know how powerful the *miasmatic disease* is. Eventually, he had been able to predict the process of what the modern biologists call immunosuppression and how immunosuppression causes perpetual immune failure. In the following lines, Hahnemann described the

---

[45] Hahnemann, *Chronic Disease*. P. 6

development of *psora* and understanding the process of the development of *psora* can help us to understand the process of the development of a *miasm* in general:

> The nerve which was first affected by the miasma has already communicated it in <u>an invisible dynamic manner</u> to the nerves of the rest of the body, and the living organism has at once, all unperceived, been so penetrated by this specific excitation, that it has been <u>compelled to appropriate this miasma</u> gradually to itself until the change of the whole being to a man thoroughly psoric, and thus the internal development of the psora, has reached completion.[46]

While explaining the development of *psora*, Hahnemann acknowledged the limitations of his observation with the phrase, 'an invisible dynamic manner'. He did not know how germs, bacteria, virus, protozoa, etc grow in human body; so he simply guessed that the miasmatic diseases grow in 'an invisible dynamic manner'. The most important thing in the development of a *miasm* is the forceful appropriation of the disease in the organism. In the abovementioned lines, Hahnemann held the power of miasmatic disease responsible for the forceful appropriation of the disease. But throughout the whole *Chronic Disease*, Hahnemann mentioned other factors such as suppressive medication, inherited deficiency to prevent the appropriation of the disease, etc which are responsible too for this appropriation. However, those homoeopaths, who are reluctant to acknowledge the role of germs in the development of *miasm*, have misunderstood Hahnemann so far grossly. Right in the next paragraph, Hahnemann explains the role of skin-eruption as an important part of the diseased *vital force*'s endeavor to fight off the disease.

> Only when the whole organism feels itself transformed by this peculiar chronic-miasmatic disease, the <u>diseased *vital force* endeavors to alleviate and to soothe the internal malady through the establishment of a suitable local symptom on the skin, the itch-vesicles</u>. So long as this eruption continues in its normal form, the internal, with its secondary ailments, cannot break forth, but must remain covered, slumbering, latent and bound.[47]

The essence of this paragraph is that since skin eruption is an essential part of the *vital force's* defense against the internal itch disease, the eruption should be there until the *vital force* can totally clear off the internal disease. Medication should be aimed at helping the *vital force* to fight with the internal disease. It should not interfere into the *vital force's* fight against the disease. Therefore, the forced omission of the eruptions by external application never cures internal

---

[46] Hahnemann, *Chronic Disease*. P. 34
[47] Hahnemann, *Chronic Disease*. P. 34

disease. Rather it interferes into the normal defense functions of the *vital force* by preventing it from doing its own job. Look, this universal utterance about the reality of the immune system of an organism was declared by a man who was born almost two hundred years before Elie Metchnikoff's discovery of phagocytes. So, why will this man be called the father of immunology? Also should we not reward this man with the noble prize posthumously? However, for Hahnemann, *miasm* was essentially one kind of immune deficiency which he claimed in Aphorism 5 of the *Organon of Medicine*:

> In addition, it will help the physician to bring about a cure if he can determine the most probable exciting cause in an acute cause and the <u>most significant phases</u> in the evolution of a chronic, long-lasting disease, enabling him to discover its underlying cause, usually a <u>chronic miasm</u>.[48]

Here, the phrase, "the <u>most significant phases</u> in the evolution of a chronic, long-lasting disease" is synonymous to "a <u>chronic miasm</u>". Yet some over-enthusiasts may wonder if *miasms* are the states of immune deficiencies, then why Hahnemann called them *contagious*? For example, in Aphorism 33 he says,

> The living human organism is far more susceptible to and disposed to be influenced by medicinal pathogenetic forces than by ordinary natural ones and <u>contagious miasms</u>. In other words, <u>*natural disease-agents*</u> *have only a subordinate and conditional, often very conditional, power to alter human health....*

It seems that despite all those endeavors to redefine, Hahnemann's *miasm* is still medieval because it passes from man to man like the medieval ones. Please note carefully the two underlined phrases, '<u>contagious miasms</u>' and '<u>*natural disease-agents*</u>'. Though Hahnemann considered *miasm* as contagious, it is the 'natural *disease-agent*s' which infect the organism. Unlike the *medieval miasma* which is supposed to infect through air, Hahnemann's *miasma* infects through contagion. In this process of contagion, the '<u>*natural disease-agents*</u>' (which is very much similar to germ) play a crucial role. Indeed, the fact whether Hahnemann belonged to the miasmatist or the contagionist group is not clear; but the use of two words, 'contagious' and 'miasm' together in the same aphorism shows that Hahnemann was less concerned about how disease spreads; rather he was more concerned about the interaction between the *vital force* and *the disease*.

There may be another reason why Hahnemann called *miasm* highly contagious. At some point of his research, Hahnemann found that almost all the patients including the patients of both sycosis and syphilis miasms suffered from the *psora* once in their life. Possibly he was troubled by the question, 'why are there so many psora patients?' He might have faced

---

[48] Hahnemann, *Organon of Medicine*. P. 34

another question. After further research on the nature of chronic disease, Hahnemann was convinced that "new ailments can result from suppression of prior ailments, which in turn, may be caused due to suppression of ailment occurring prior to it. This process of 'suppression of disease' was a common observation of many physicians including Hahnemann."[49] So for Hahnemann, the suppression of *psora* occurs into *sycosis* and the suppression of *sycosis* occurs into *syphilis*. But he was most probably confronted with the question: how does *psora* occur? At this point, he guessed that *psora* is so much contagious that a patient may contract it "perhaps already in the cradle, or communicated in some other unrecallable fashion". If he knew that a man genetically inherits a part of his parents' *vital force* (or immune defense) and vital deficiency (immune deficiency), he would possibly replace the phrase, 'in some other unrecallable fashion' with 'by birth'.

---

[49] Mathur. "The concept of miasm—evolution and present day perspective"

4
HAHNEMANN'S *DISEASE-AGENT* EQUIVALENT TO *GERMS*? WHAT IS *MIASM* THEN REALLY?

For Hahnemann, disease is not any external material force; rather it is internal and mostly the reaction of the *vital force* (the *vital force*'s ways of speaking off the disturbance caused by the *dynamic influence* of the hostile *disease-agent*). Rather for him, disease is the state of *untuneness* of the *vital force* which is caused by "outer malefic agents that harm the healthy organism and disturb the harmonious rhythm of life can reach and affect the spirit-like dynamis only in a way that also is dynamic and spirit-like".[50] So, *miasm* is, as it is traditionally believed, not the cause of *disease*; rather Hahnemann believed that some *disease-agent* or *outer malefic agents* cause the *untuneness* or the *disease* of *vital force*. In order to understand what *miasm* really is, one must not confuse the terms *disease*, *disease-agent* and *miasm* with each other. Hahnemann knew nothing about germs. But he was aware of something which causes *disease*. He used the term *disease-agent* to denote this cause of disease. Certainly, there is a very sophisticated but crucial difference between this *disease-agent* and *miasm*. Please note in the following statement of Hahnemann, where *disease* and *disease-agent* are two different things:

> When man falls ill it is at first only this self-sustaining spirit-like *vital force* (vital principle) everywhere present in the organism which is untuned by the *dynamic influence* of the hostile *disease-agent*. It is only this *vital force* thus untuned which brings about in the organism the disagreeable sensations and abnormal functions that we call disease.[51]

Here, in the footnote of this aphorism, Hahnemann refers to two distinct

---

[50] Samuel Hahneman, Organon of Medicine, Para-16
[51] Samuel Hahneman, Organon of Medicine, Para-11

factors: a. *disease* and b. *disease-agent*. He has no interest in "finding causative factors for acute infectious diseases inside the body of the patients".[52] If we consider the *disease-agent* as an undiscoverable factor X and its *dynamic influence* as function Y, like many others of his contemporaries, Hahnemann also provided explanations of the *disease-agent* X and its *dynamic influence* as function Y in the following manner: "just as a child with small pox or measles communicates to a near, untouched healthy child in a invisible manner (dynamically) the small pox or measles, that is, infect it at a distance without anything from the infective child going or capable of going to the one to be infected."[53] I will not say anything about whether it is scientific or not. Rather, in my opinion, it never falsifies the validity of Hahnemann's epoch-making discovery of the *vital power* (immune system). I think, Hahnemann's discovery of the *vital power* (not in medieval sense) is as important as his 'like cures like' theory. Moreover, it helps us to make clear distinctions among *disease, disease-agent, dynamic influence* and *miasm*. Look you must keep in mind that the *dynamic influence* of the *disease-agent* and *miasm* are two distinct subjects, though most of the homoeopaths fail to perceive the difference between them. The way how Mohit Mathur (2009) perceived *miasm* in the following sentence is an error which most of the homoeopaths commit: "*To explain the mechanism of spread of these acute miasms among people he wrote, explaining the term 'dynamic influence' in the footnote to the 11th aphorism of the Organon*".[54] How does this author claim that, in Aphorism 11, Hahnemann explained "the mechanism of spread of these acute miasms"? Read again between the lines of the footnote of Aphorism 11:

> What is dynamic influence, dynamic force? We see that the earth causes the moon to revolve around it in twenty-eight days and a number of hours by some invisible mysterious force…
>
> In the same way, the dynamic force with which pathogenetic influences act on healthy individuals and the dynamic force with which medicines act upon the vital principle to restore health are nothing but a contagion devoid of any material or mechanical aspect. A magnet powerfully attracts a piece of iron or steel near it in a similar way…….
>
> In a similar way a child who has smallpox or measles will transmit them to a healthy child by approaching him, even without touching him. This contamination takes place invisibly (dynamically) at a distance, with no more transmission of any material particle from one to the other than from the magnet to the steel needle. A specific, spirit-like influence

---

[52] Mohit Mathur. "The concept of miasm—evolution and present day perspective", Homeopathy (2009) 98, 177–180
[53] Samuel Hahneman, *Organon of Medicine*, Para-11
[54] Mohit Mathur. "The concept of miasm—evolution and present day perspective", Homeopathy (2009) 98, 177–180

communicates smallpox or measles to the child nearby, just as the magnet communicates magnetic force to the needle.[55]

You will see that the whole footnote is, indeed, an explanation of the *dynamic influence* of the *disease-agent*. Hahnemann provided the example of the process of how small pox or measles transmits from an affected child to a healthy one. Does it mean that the *miasm* spreads from person to another through contagion? Or does it mean that the *disease-agent* spreads through the magnet like *dynamic influence* after contagion? In the second half of the preceding chapter, I have shown the whole process of the development of *miasm* which Hahnemann described in the *Chronic Disease*. Please take a look at it again:

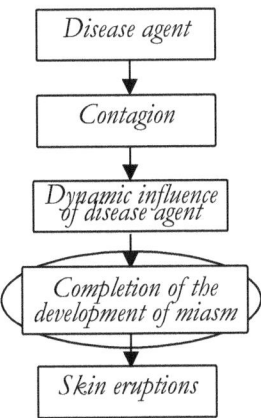

Here, we will try to prove Hahnemann's *miasm* is different from medieval *miasma* in the sense that the first one is fundamentally internal state of the immune system whereas the later is some external malady which infects people from time to time through air. Suppose Mr. Y has been infected with pox. First he came into contact with *disease-agent* of pox. The *disease-agent* of pox starts influencing the organism dynamically and the *miasm* of pox grew through the affection of the inner whole of Mr. Y. Finally, eruptions of pox show on skin. Now, if we consider Mr. Mohit Mathur's claim (that *miasm* itself spreads through dynamic influence) true, it falsifies the role of Hahnemann's *disease-agent* in the development of the *untuned state* of *vital force* and *miasm*, because in such case (if we consider that *miasm* itself spreads), the process of infection does not need any *disease-agent*. But the '*disease-agent*' is a very crucial

---

[55] Samuel Hahneman, *Organon of Medicine*, Para-73

step in the process of the development of *miasm*, as Hahnemann acknowledges:

> The psychic and physical inimical influences that we encounter in the world and that we call *disease-agent*s do not have an absolute power to untune our organism. We fall ill under their influence only when the organism is disposed and susceptible enough to their attack for its feelings and function to be altered and untuned from the normal. Thus these *disease-agent*s do not make everybody sick each time.[56]

Referring to Aphorism73, Mohit Mathoor claimed, "Hahnemann used the term 'acute miasm' for all such acute infectious <u>diseases</u>."[57] If the underlined word '<u>disease</u>' is taken according to Hahnemann's definition of *disease*, it is true that diseases like small pox, measles, etc cause short-time untuned or sickness of the *vital force*, and the *vital force* gets the upper-hand quickly if it is not maltreated by suppressive medications and not conditioned by other miasms (or *untuneness* or immune deficiency). But if '<u>disease</u>' is taken in its traditional sense, Mathoor's perception of Hahnemann's *miasm* is miserably wrong. He claims that Hahnemann's *miasm* (acute in this context) spreads like infectious diseases through contagion. But such claim is essentially the affirmation of that Hahnemann's *miasm* is essentially the medieval one. But in reality it is very much different from the medieval one.

Hahnemann's *miasm* is neither the counterpart of infectious disease-agent nor the medieval miasma concept. Read Aphorism73; it begins as following: "There are acute diseases affecting single individuals, diseases brought on by harmful influences to which particular individuals have been exposed".[58] The phrase, '<u>diseases brought on by harmful influences</u>', implies that *diseases* are brought on by harmful influences [of *disease-agent*]. Does it mean that 'harmful influence [of *disease-agent*]' is equal to the term '*acute miasm*'? Is *miasm* any external force as Mohit Mathur imagined? Or is it an internal state of man? So, it is clear that Hahnemann's *miasm* does not spread as Mohit Mathur claimed. It is not infectious as Dr. Timothy Decker and others imagined. It does not cause *disease*; rather it is the diseased state (of the *vital force*) which fails to prevent disease. It does not have any *dynamic or harmful influence* because Hahnemann says that *dynamic or harmful influence* is the property of *disease-agent*. Then what is *miasm*? Let's explore into Hahnemann's writings in order to find what it is.

ARE MIASMS THE STAGES OF IMMUNE DEFICIENCY?

Wherever Hahnemann mentioned about *miasm* in his writings, he did so

---

[56] Samuel Hahneman, Organon of Medicine, Para-31
[57] Mohit Mathur. "The concept of miasm—evolution and present day perspective", Homeopathy (2009) 98, 177–180
[58] Samuel Hahneman, Organon of Medicine, Para-73

necessarily in an attempt to explain the recurrence of *disease*. The very essence of *miasm* is that it has a direct or indirect connection to *diseases* which are chronic. Hahnemann did not make any attempt to prove *miasm* through any scientific method. Rather he theorized it from his empirical evidences and in most cases, he described *miasm* without referring to any example and showing the logical processes which assisted him in reaching the conclusions which he made about miasm. So, *miasm* was an unknown factor X which Hahnemann brooded on and endeavored to induce conclusions for. Let's decode Hahnemann's perception about *miasm* in order for understanding what X stands for. We will further see if there is any modern biological equivalent to Hahnemann's *miasm* or X.

The very first statement about *miasm* that comes in Aphorism 5 of the Organon of Medicine affirms that chronic *miasm* is an underlying cause of a chronic, long-lasting *disease*. Earlier in this article, I proved that *miasm* is not any material cause of *disease* like Hahnemann's concept of *disease-agent*. So, what type of underlying cause is it? Hahnemann says that untuned *vital force* is the cause of *disease*. Does not it mean that *miasm*, the underlying cause of a chronic, long-lasting *disease*, is the long-term *untuneness* of *vital force*? Numerous lines from the *Organon of Medicine* show that *vital power* (in healthy state) has the tendency and ability to stay tuned. So *miasm*, the underlying cause of a chronic long-lasting *disease*, is the long-term failure of the *vital force* to stay tuned. So when Hahnemann tells about acute *miasm* in Aphorism 73, he necessarily means the short-term immune-failures which are caused by germs of seasonal infectious diseases such "smallpox, measles, whooping cough, the old, bright red, smooth scarlatina of Sydenham, mumps, etc".[59] The same Aphorism proves that Hahnemann was aware of the *vital force*'s lifelong ability to defend against those seasonal infectious germs, if contracted for once in lifetime. So, when Hahnemann tells about contagious *miasm* (Aphorism 33), he necessarily refers to the short-term 'immune failures' (*vital force*'s failure to stay tuned) which are caused by contagious germs. Furthermore, Hahnemann was the first to notice the evolution of *miasm* or *immune failure*.

> In addition, it will help the physician to bring about a cure if he can determine the most probable exciting cause in an acute cause and the most significant phases in the evolution of a chronic, long-lasting disease, enabling him to discover its underlying cause, usually a chronic miasm.

Hahnemann was the first who was ever to tell about chronic immune failure and to notice the phases of the evolution of *immune failure*. He believed that *miasm* or chronic immune failure may start from the suppression of acute diseases. Obviously the beginning phase of the evolution of *miasm* is *Psora* which is later followed by *Sycosis* and then *Syphilis*. We have already learnt that

---

[59] Samuel Hahneman, *Organon of Medicine*, Para-73

Hahnemann's *miasm* is essentially the immune failure or the failure of *vital force* to stay tuned. So Hahnemann's attempt to divide *miasm* into three phases *Psora*, *Sycosis* and *Syphilis* is essentially his attempt to assess the phases of immune failure of a patient's *vital force*. There are ample scientific evidences and proofs that show that Hahnemann's *Psora-Sycosis-Syphilis* sequence represents the essence of the progression of the immune-diseases. In order for knowing how Hahnemann's *miasm* sequence bears the essence of the progression of the modern immune-diseases, we need to look at the whole disease-mechanism:

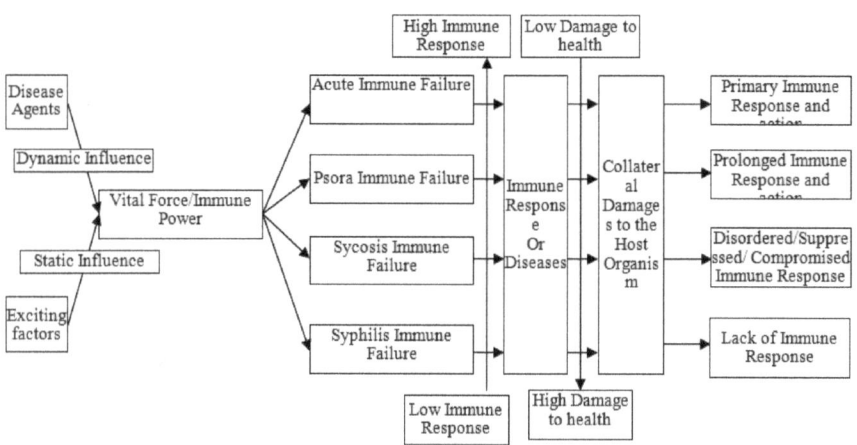

CAUSES OF DISEASE: IMMUNE DEFICIENCY (*MIASM*) OR *GERMS*?

The above diagram of disease-progress is essentially Hahnemann's concept of *disease* and its progress. I can quote innumerable lines from the *Organon of Medicine* and *Chronic Diseases* in support of the logical construction of this diagram. According to Hahnemann, *disease* is essentially a matter of the *vital force*. Hence, *disease-agents* with *dynamic influence* are necessarily the catalysts of the aggravation of the health of the host organisms. Here, *dynamic influence* should be assessed as the ability of the *disease-agents* to be lethal to the organisms. So, the immune response or the response of the *vital force* to the *disease-agents* will vary according to its *miasms*. Here, we can consider the following:

$$Vital\ force \approx Dynamic\ influence\ of\ Disease\text{-}agents$$
$$Or,\ Vital\ force > Dynamic\ influence\ of\ Disease\text{-}agents\ (in\ health)$$
$$Or,\ Vital\ force < Dynamic\ influence\ of\ Disease\text{-}agents\ (in\ disease)$$

Ideally, in health, the *vital force* is in a winning state. It does not mean that it will never fall ill. It means that the *vital force* is in continuous struggle with external material and organic threats; the *vital force* is sturdy enough to slaughter most of the threats at great ease and it becomes stressed to annihilate few of them. So, it may suffer from fever, cough, cold, etc from time to time. In winning state, exposure to external threats cannot cause much damage to the *vital force* unless the *vital force* is in a situation which causes damages to the *vital force*. Thus, the Psora (primary immune failure) *miasm* starts. Maltreatment, suppression, long-term exposure to malignant forces and genetic inheritance play the most crucial role in the development of Psora. *Vital force* (immune system) with Psoriatic flaws cannot heal on its own because of the defects within the immune system itself. So, the Psora starts the deteriorations of the organs and organisms which are involved in the preservation of the health and the immune system itself; it means *miasm* destroys the *vital force* itself. Though very few Homeopaths are aware of this trait of miasm, almost none of them know how *miasm* destroys it. Hahnemann explains this whole process in Aphorism 73:

> The others, insignificant and often unnoticed at the beginning, dynamically untune the living organism, each in its own way, and remove it from health gradually, in such a way that the automatic vital energy (*vital force*, vital principle) intended for the preservation of health can offer only imperfect, inappropriate, ineffective resistance to them, both at their start and as they continue, and can never extinguish them; on its own with its own power, so that it must impotently let them flourish while it becomes ever more untuned, until the organism is finally destroyed. We call these chronic diseases; they arise from the dynamic contagion of a chronic miasm.[60]

This is why Hahnemann keeps *Psora* at the beginning of the deterioration of the immune system. When the immune system fails to build successful resistance to malignant forces, it starts to become affected by those forces. So, it becomes disordered and deranged. The outcome of this disorder is obvious. The immune system grows abnormal and fails to differentiate between the 'self' and the 'non-self' organisms. Hahnemann marked this abnormality of the immune system as the excesses of the mind, body and *vital force* (immune system). This abnormally behaving *vital force* (immune system) further becomes complicated with the progressing deterioration of the immunity organs. Ultimately, the immune system loses its ability to respond against external malignant forces. For Hahnemann, this phase of the deterioration of the *vital force* (immune system) is Syphilis. How much scientific is such sequence of the deterioration of the *vital force* (immune system)? Look at the following:

---

[60] Samuel Hahneman, *Organon of Medicine*, Para-73

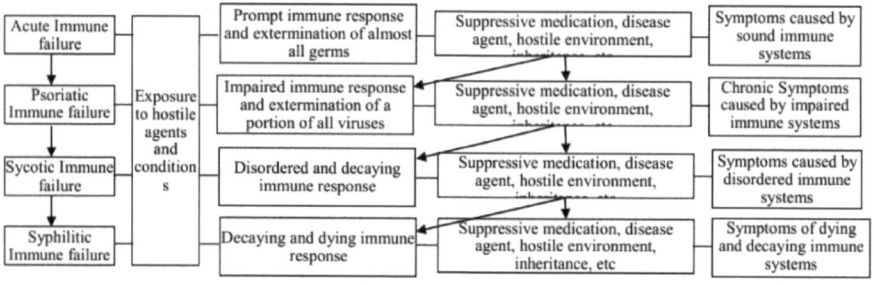

AN EXPERIMENT: EFFECTS OF GERMS ON PEOPLE WITH DIFFERENT IMMUNE ABILITIES

Hahnemann's attempt to view *disease* as the Transition or evolution of the immune system is quite scientific and, at the same time, it is a revolt against the allopaths' attempt to view the roots of diseases in germs and to invest billions of dollars in developing strategies and chemical poisons to kill those germs. If the same germs do not affect different people with different immune abilities in the same ways, are the germs alone the cause of disease? This question was asked by Hahnemann almost 250 years ago and it has remained still relevant today. For Hahnemann, disease is not an "entity....separate from its living totality; or and entity separate from the *vital force*, from the dynamic power that gives life to the organism".[61] In *Chronic Disease*, Hahnemann further claims that the same virus of hydrophobia does not affect all victims in the same way:

> Among many persons bitten by mad dogs—thanks to the benign ruler of the world—only few are infected, rarely the twelfth; often, as I myself have observed, only one out of twenty or thirty persons bitten. The others, even if ever so badly mangled by the mad dog, usually all recover, even if they are not treated by a physician or surgeon.[62]

The allopaths' tendency of ignoring the roll of the immune system in cure and the fallacy of curing a disease by killing the germs can be proved futile in the following experiment. Obviously the experiment should focus on the

---

[61] Samuel Hahneman, *Organon of Medicine*, Para-13
[62] Samuel Hahneman, *Chronic Diseases*. P. 34

question if the same pernicious pathogen X affects all the persons, P, Q, R, S (having different immune states respectively as Acute, Psora, Sycosis, Syphilis) with the same degree of severity. Imagine as following:

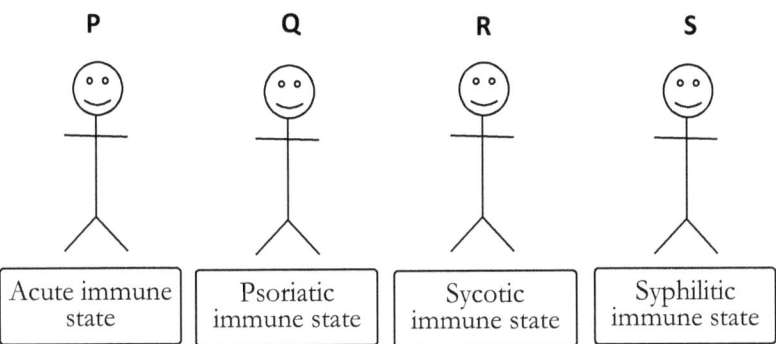

If the pathogen X (here we assume that the amount of X is below the lethality index) is injected into all the four persons P, Q, R and S, what will be their immune responses to it? In the case of P, we will assume that P does not suffer from any of the Psoriatic, Sycotic and Syphilitic immune failures. So, the P's protection against Xs will be the highest and suffering from the symptoms will be within the shortest possible timeframe. Without medication, P's immune system will recover on its own protecting its immune organs quite well.

Now, the immune system of Q will take longer time (than P takes) to develop resistance against the germs X. This inability of Psora person Q to develop resistance against this germ is engendered by various factors such as suppressive medication, virility of *disease-agent*, person's behavior, lifestyle, hostile environment, inheritance, etc. in this state, the immune system is quite sound and sturdy, though its activities and functions are interfered, hindered and suppressed by the aforementioned factors. The virility of the germs could do almost nothing to the important organs of the body.

Since the person R has reached the Sycotic state, it underwent all the hostile factors which the Psora patients normally suffer from. However, it has already yielded and compromised to the pressure and suppression, and grown confusion of its functions and duties. It is now disordered and disarranged. It does not know what to defend, and when to take offense. When the germs X are injected, R's immune responses are scattered, disordered and confused. So, the germs can cause maximum damages to the important organs (including the immune system organs). Further suppression and other aforementioned factors gradually will take R's immune system to the Syphilitic state.

Now, S's immune power is in Syphilitic state and it already underwent the ruinations at the Psora and Sycotic stages. In this stage, the immune system organs are decaying and dying. There is not effective defense against the germs. They are destroying the host cells freely and merciless triumph. So, the cells are rotting and melting down.

Here, what should be the possible treatment strategies for these four persons to get rid of the sufferings? Since modern immunology says that sufferings are the natural response of the immune systems to threats, they should not be suppressed or compromised. No painkiller or anything which suppresses the immune functions should be used to get rid of the symptoms. So, we have one reasonable goal of exterminating the germs in order to get rid of the sufferings which are caused by germs X. It is to exterminate the germs and to restore the health to its earlier state so that the patient needs to depend on the medicine as less as possible.

We will see if simply killing germs X with antibiotics helps us achieve this goal of curing the patient. Antibiotics are popularly used to kill or prevent the growth of harmful bacteria. Almost all of the medical literatures tell about the use of antibiotics for bacterial infections; but when the antibiotics fail to prevent infection, they blame either the selection of antibiotics or the resistance of the bacteria to antibiotics. These authors will never mention the most important roles of the immune system in curing the infection. They will not consider if the patient's immune system is in a state to take the privileges of antibiotics. There is every possibility that what they blame as drug-resistance or wrong selection of antibiotics is indeed the patient's immune failure to fight back invading germs (as Hahnemann speculated). How do they ignore the functions of immune systems which comprise a big scenario in cure? For viral infections, medical scholars acknowledge that immune system play the main part in healing, as it is said in Medicineplus: "For most viral infections, treatments can only help with symptoms while you wait for your immune system to fight off the virus".[63] Look what Adam Felman says about the role of immune system in healing viral infection: "Most treatment aims to relieve symptoms while the immune system combats the virus without assistance from medicine".[64] Indeed, these statements denote two factors regarding healing: first, healing with the assistance of medicines; second, healing backed by immune system itself. Now the question is: if the immune system does not have the ability to heal on its own, what is the use of antibiotics in bacterial infection? Can antibiotics really cure a Sycotic or a Syphilitic patient whose immune system has been deranged or dying? Here

---

[63] Medicineplus. "Viral Infections", US National Library of Medicine. https://medlineplus.gov/viralinfections.html

[64] Adam Felman. "Everything you need to know about infections", Medical News Today. https://www.medicalnewstoday.com/articles/196271.php

starts Allopaths' lifelong palliative care for the patients whom the Homoeopaths consider as Sycotic and Syphilitic.

So, if a child of 7 or 8 years suffers from Asthma and cold allergy (or any of such chronic diseases) what he/she inherits from his/her parents, he/she will be prescribed with one from tons of leukotriene receptor antagonists and antihistamines for life-time. It is because this child has inherited Sycosis from his parents. Along the passage of time, he/she will depend more and more on more powerful drugs. Possibly during his adulthood, this child will not be but a living corpse who will pass his first wedding night with an inhaler. Is there any effective solution to this miserable condition? Unless the immune system does not have the ability to roll back to its healthy state, permanent cure is impossible with the assistance of allopathic drugs. So, in allopathic medical sector, there is no light of hope for this child of Sycotic immune state.

But Hahnemann's attempt to discover homoeopathy was an outright rebellion against the despair which the allopathic medical system lets a patient plunge into. In the very first place, he defies the allopathic practices of using chemicals as suppressors of symptoms, declaring that a doctor's goal is to restore a patient or a patient's *vital force* (or his immune system) to health. He must not suppress the patient's symptoms because such suppression will result into derangement and confusion of the patients' *vital force* (immune system) which will lead him to a Sycotic state. Hahnemann vehemently opposed modern allopathic quackery (of suppressing the immune system) which Adam Felman expressed so naively in the following statement: "Most treatment aims to relieve symptoms while the immune system………………"[65] He further claimed that 'treatment according to the similarity of symptoms' will necessarily assist the immune system to roll back nearer to its healthy state. Indeed, Hahnemann's claim "Like cures like" was an epoch-making statement. Like most of Hahnemann's concepts i.e. vital power, *miasm*, suppression, etc, 'like cures like' is another concept which was even more complex for the people of his era. He advocated this idea to people who knew nothing about the immune system. Also Hahnemann did not have any scientific proofs of immune system of human body. But his reasoning and observations assisted him to conceive the idea of *vital force* which is nearer to the idea of modern immune system than any other concept in the history of medical science.

---

[65] Adam Felman. "Everything you need to know about infections",

5
HOMOEOPATHY: AN OVERNIGHT DISCOVERY? HOW MUCH CREDIBLE IS THE STORY OF CINCHONA?

Do you think that Hahnemann's Homoeopathy is an overnight discovery? Please go through the Organon of Medicine, you will see that almost one-third of the book tells about what is the role of *vital force* in human body, why and how *vital force* produces disease, what *miasm* is, how suppression occurs with dissimilar medicines, why a physician should treat the man (or *vital force* or immune system), not the disease, etc. Have you noticed why Hahnemann spent so much of his effort to explain these concepts? Why did he not simply tell "disease should be cured only by those that can artificially produce similar disease symptoms"?[66] Hahnemann certainly was aware of the pathogenic effects of his claimed-medicines on human body. If a substance produces some artificial diseases, how could he claim that the same substance will cure the same natural diseases? Apparently, such claim is insane, illogical and paradoxical. Why would he make such an apparently idiotic comment which would turn him into a laughingstock? Do you think that Hahnemann claimed it whimsically without any reasoning or any logic? No! It was Hahnemann's well-thought and decisive claim which is quite coherent with his version of immune system (*vital force*, which he describes so ardently in almost one-third of the Organon of Medicine) and with the modern immune system also. For Hahnemann, *vital force* is indeed a self-protective intelligent, autocratic and complicated defense system of the body. Symptoms such as pain, inflammation, itching, cough, mucous, swellings, heat, etc are visible aftermaths of the *vital force*'s internal protective activities. Let consider the following scenarios in order to understand how Homoeopathy and Allopathy cures a patient:

Suppose, a patient P is suffering from viral flu with itching, fever or feeling

---

[66] Samuel Hahneman, Organon of Medicine, Para-71

feverish/chills, cough, sore throat, runny nose, muscle aches, headache, fatigue, vomiting and diarrhea. We will try to know the comparative mechanism of actions of allopathic and homoeopathic medicines which this patient needs to come round within the shortest possible time.

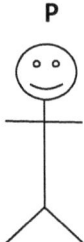

Suffering from viral flu (or bacterial infection) with itches, fever or feeling feverish/chills, cough, sore throat, runny nose, muscle aches, headache, fatigue, vomiting and diarrhea

Let's see why your body produces these symptoms. Modern immunology says that almost all the symptoms play very important roles in instigating immune responses against any virulent agents, forces or diseases. If a human body fails to produce any of the symptoms, it is possible that it will not be able to start proper immune defense against the invading disease-agents. Researchers have discovered a direct regulatory relationship between the nervous system and the immune defense. It is believed that "the CNS controls the immune system through several pathways, among them hardwired fibres of the autonomic nervous system".[67] The sensory receptors which are spread

---

[67] Brommer B, Engel O, Kopp MA, Watzlawick R, Müller S, Prüss H, Chen Y, DeVivo MJ, Finkenstaedt FW, Dirnagl U, Liebscher T, Meisel A, Schwab JM. Spinal cord injury-induced immune deficiency syndrome enhances infection susceptibility dependent on lesion level. Brain. 2016 Jan 10. https://www.ncbi.nlm.nih.gov/pmc/articles/PMC5014125/

over the whole body maintain a realtime connection between the nervous system and the immune organs. The brain is continually updated by the peripheral nervous system about the immune status of the body and subsequent counter measures are taken to annihilate any possible threats. Obviously symptoms are the results of the interactions between the immune system and the nervous system. Look at the following how a body produces symptoms:

Steps in the Inflammatory Response

- **histamine**
  - Allow: Blood vessels to dilate, become more permeable & allow more Defense cells to the wound area
- 3 parts of the inflammation responses?
- 1. Blood Vessels dilate
  - heat
- 2. leaky capillaries:
  - Pain & Swelling (aka: edema)
- 3. NEUTROPHILS ENTER BLOOD FROM BONE MARROW AND GO TOWARDS CHEMICAL "SCENT"
  - SQUEEZE THROUGH THE CAPILLARY WALL (DIAPEDESIS)
  - NEUTROPHILS GATHER AT SPOT OF TISSUE INJURY. EAT FOREIGN MATERIALS
  - PHAGOCYTES COME LATER- turn into MACROPHAGES (eating machines)
- Pus indicates a possible problem.

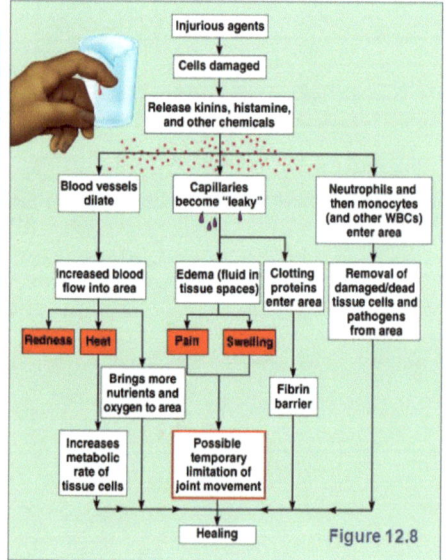

Figure: Steps in immune response[68]

---

[68] Image collected from internet

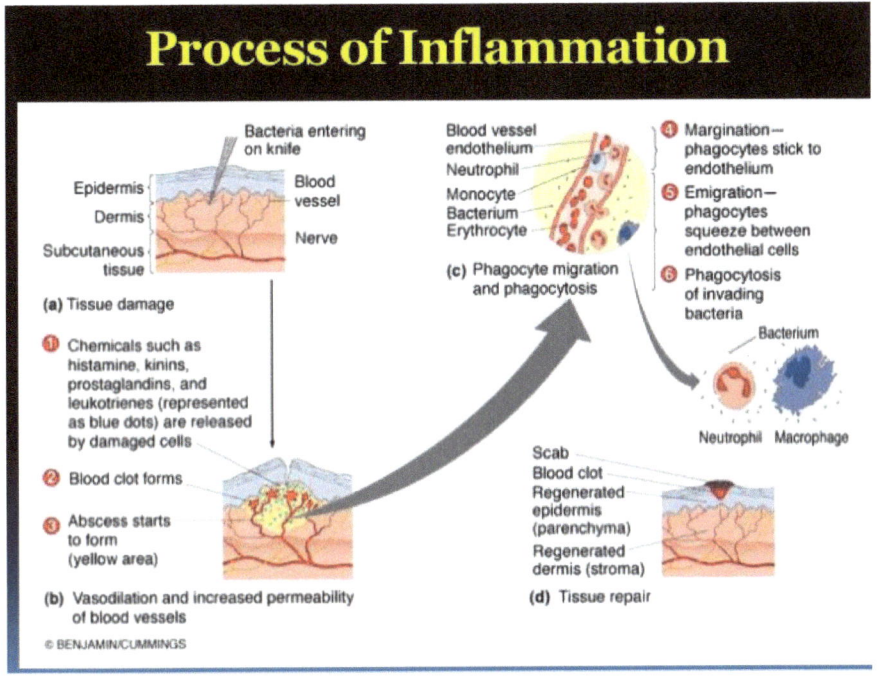

Figure: Process of inflammation[69]

The abovementioned picture of the steps of immune-responses is quite self-explanatory. The symptoms like itches, fever, cough, nose-run, etc play the roles of igniters of further immune responses. For example, release of histamine by the damaged cells causes itching which is unpleasant for the patient, but histamines are important for increasing the blood-flow (as a result of vasodilatation) to the damaged area for increased immune-performances such as heat generation, causing inflammation, increasing metabolic rate of cells, bringing neutrophils to the site of injury to kill and deactivate the pathogens and other immune-responses. Furthermore, the secretion of cytokines by macrophages signals path to injury site and initiates tissue-repair. So, it is clear that each of the symptoms has their own specific functions which are responsible for a number of subsequent immune-responses. Let's make a list:

---

[69] Image collected from internet

Histamine/Prostaglandin
Symptoms:
Itching, runny nose, watery eyes,
inflammation, redness, swelling, etc

Vasodilatation for increasing blood-flow

Calling neutrophils for killing foreign bodies

Increased permeability of blood vessels for allowing neutrophils and macrophages to pass into the site of affections

Playing some roles in producing heat for increasing metabolic rate of cells

THE SCIENCE OF HOMOEOPATHIC IMMUNOLOGY

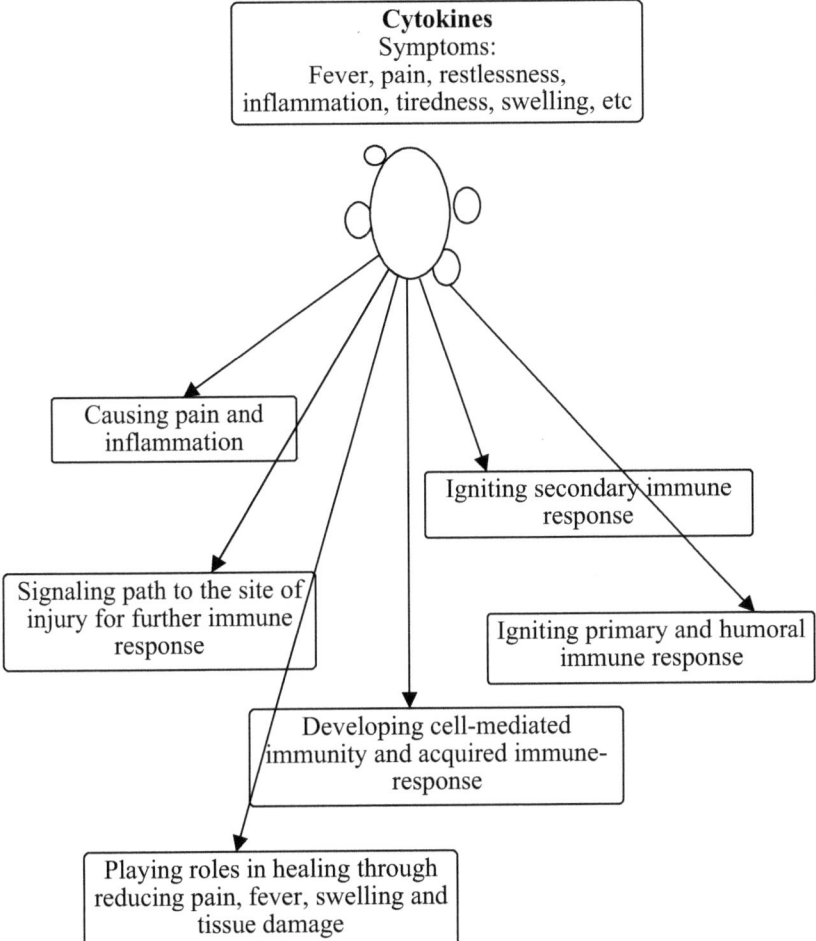

The abovementioned two figures are, indeed, our futile attempts to explain symptoms and immune-response relations. It is almost impossible to write down all the symptoms and their subsequent roles in immune-response within few pages without annoying the readers. The symptoms of our patient P definitely show that his immune-system is struggling earnestly to fight off the invading germs. Since the germs are virulent, the symptoms are overwhelming. According to allopathic view, the symptoms of this patient can be mitigated with the aid of so-called modern medicines within minutes. These medicines are so effective that they will arrest the secretions of the villains (with merciless triumph) who are responsible for so much pains and sufferings of the patient. Which villains do these medicines act against? Suppose that Ibuprofen has been prescribed to this patient. It is a "medication in the non-steroidal anti-inflammatory drug (NSAID) class that is used for treating pain, fever, and inflammation". It suppresses the "production of prostaglandins, substances that the body releases in response to illness and injury".[70] Now, it is clear that Prostaglandins are those villains who unnecessarily (?) and villainously (?) throw the patients into utmost pains and sufferings. Take a look at what villainy the prostaglandins do to the patients and why they inflict so much suffering. Indeed, prostaglandins are hormone-like chemical compounds that are responsible for a number of important physical functions such as vasodilatation of vascular smooth muscles, causing aggregation and disaggregation of platelets, sensitizing spinal neurons to pain, inducing labor, regulating intraocular pressure, regulating inflammation, regulating calcium movement and hormones, controlling cell-growth, acts on hypothalamus to produce fever, regulating glomerulus filtration rate, controlling acid secretion through parietal cells of stomach, controlling uterine contraction during menstruation and thousands of other known and unknown functions which directly or indirectly related to the healthy functioning of the immune systems. Indeed, the production of prostaglandins is a part of the signaling system of a man's immune defense. The most crucial defense functions of the immune system entail the production of prostaglandins. So, if your body produces prostaglandins in response to infection, your immune systems will take instant offenses and subsequent defensive actions. Ibuprofen stops the productions of prostaglandins in order to relieve the patients from pain, fever, inflammation, etc. But does it cure you from the infections? Will you shut your watchdog's mouth up in order to sleep well at night? Read the lines from Wikipedia: "Ibuprofen is a medication in the non-steroidal anti-inflammatory drug (NSAID) class that is used for treating (?) pain, fever, and inflammation".[71] Please take a look at the big lie which a popular website like Wikipedia is selling among the innocent readers. Does Ibuprofen treat "pain,

---

[70] C. Fookes. "Nonsteroidal anti-inflammatory drugs", Drugs. https://www.drugs.com/drug-class/nonsteroidal-anti-inflammatory-agents.html
[71] Wikipedia. "Ibuprufen", https://en.wikipedia.org/wiki/Ibuprofen

fever, and inflammation"? Or does it dodge the immune system? If you have a burglar-alarm and if it becomes activated every midnight, what will be the solution? Will you cut off its electricity supply so that it stops disturbing your sleep? Or will you take necessary steps to arrest the thief?

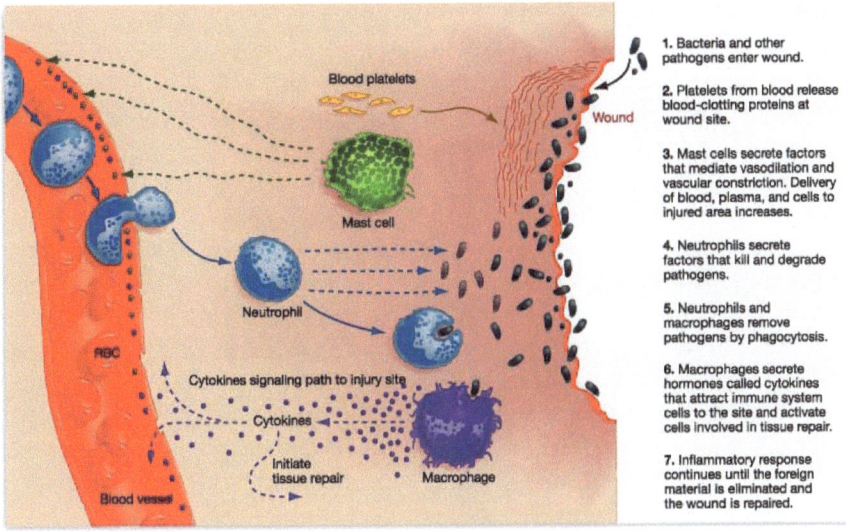

Figure: Process of immune responses[72]

Hahnemann vehemently opposed this absolute madness of letting the patient to pass some peaceful and painless nights by turning off the natural alarming system of his immune-defense system. For him, the abovementioned way of treating (?) symptoms was the dissimilar method of treatment. The term "dissimilar way of treatment" is fraught with a number of modern immunological concepts. It necessarily connotes that this treatment method involves prescribing something as medicine which arrests or prevents the natural symptoms productions ability of the immune system. Since symptoms are the languages of the diseased immune system, suppressing them with the help of chemical compound never cures the disease. Rather long-term suppression of the immune-response compels the patient's immune system to

---

[72] Image collected from internet

assume a compromised and disordered behavior which Hahnemann called Sycotic and Syphilitic states. So, if you are not allowed to interfere into the functions of the immune system with suppressive medicines, how will the patients be cured of the sufferings? In the most parts of the "Organon of Medicine", Hahnemann describes why not to interfere into the defense functions of the *vital force* and how to cure the sufferings without such interferences. No other scholar before Hahnemann in human history preached the idea of treating the patients without intimidating the *vital force* or 'immune system'. All of the imperatives (except one, maintaining non-interference criteria) which Hahnemann advised for a physician to cure a patient are easily comprehensible. Though such pioneer attempt to build up a solid philosophical ground for medical practices should have win a prestigious position in the history of medical science, Hahnemann (despite) has been denied that position for two reasons: first, his 'like cures like' philosophy failed to receive an laboratory proof (I think, such lack of laboratory proof has been engendered by the apparently paradoxical nature of the statement), secondly, no sincere effort has ever been made to perform any laboratory test to prove the statement, since scholarly acknowledgement of homoeopathy is tremendously threatening to the existing medical industry.

I have told earlier that the version of *vital force* which Hahnemann advocated was very difficult for his contemporary scholars to grab. Despite this difficulty, Hahnemann will not be remembered for his 'like cure like' theory ('similar cure similar') so much as for his philosophy of 'vital power'. I do not know how the story of Cinchona made it place in the history of Homoeopathy. 'Like cures like' was not Hahnemann's sole discovery. Rather what is laudable in Hahnemann's attempt is to explain it from biological and medical point-of-view and to place this principle (Law of Similar) on a solid philosophical ground. (I believe someone concocted the story of Cinchona in order to establish Homoeopathy as a sudden miraculous discovery like Newton's apple or Madam Kurri's X-ray. Indeed, such stories are meant for satisfying the commoners' hunger for a cheap and easily palatable gossip which helped them to keep aside the heavy painful burden of philosophical thoughts behind the invention.)

Please note that 'like cures like' is a millennia-old observation which dated back to Hippocrates. Indeed, Hahnemann was the first man (in human history) who attempted to explain why 'cure with similar' is better than 'cure with dissimilar' and his effort resulted into the birth of *vital force*, the philosophical abstract of what modern science calls 'immune system'. Hahnemann developed this philosophy based on his observations and made sincere effort to convince his readers. But it is very much crucial how we understand it. Earlier in this paper, I have tried to dissolve a number of such misperceptions of Homeopathic concepts such as *vital force*, vitalism, 'treat the man not the disease', etc. Hahnemann's 'like-cure-like' is one of such popularly misunderstood concepts. Look at the three quotations taken from different websites:

> Hahnemann believed that if a patient had an illness, it could be cured by giving a medicine which, if given to a healthy person, would produce similar symptoms of that same illness but to a slighter degree. Thus, if a patient was suffering from severe nausea, he was given a medicine which in a healthy person would provoke mild nausea.[73]

> The law of similar is the concept that has given its name to homeopathy, which is therapy that cures a disease using the substance that can induce the same symptoms in a healthy individual (in contrast to allopathy, which is the treatment that uses opposite principles to interfere with or block pathologic processes). [74]

> Homeopathy or homeopathy is a system of alternative medicine created in 1796 by Samuel Hahnemann, based on his doctrine of like cures like (similia similibus curentur), a claim that a substance that causes the symptoms of a disease in healthy people would cure similar symptoms in sick people. [75]

In all the three abovementioned quotations, the authors have tried to convey the essence of Homoeopathy in a way which is misleading and partial. Indeed these are the perceptions of laypeople who have failed to grab the essence of Hahnemann's *vital force*. If Homoeopathy means prescribing a medicine for symptoms which the medicine itself can produce, why would Hahnemann prescribe Silicea for the intrusion of any foreign substance into human body? Does Silicea produce pus in healthy body? Whoever wrote the lines about Homoeopathy in Wikipedia is no one but an inert layperson who, because of his intellectual incapability to perceive the complex mechanism of Hahnemann's *vital force*, needs an easy outlet "Like cures like". Indeed, 'like cure like' or the abovementioned quotations never represent even a little part of Homoeopathy. If it were the primary concern of Hahnemann, why did he spend much of his precious effort to explain *vital force* and its complex mechanisms in the Organon of Medicine? Indeed, the abovementioned mentioned perceptions about Homoeopathy are compatible with Hahnemann's explanation of how the medicinal substances cure the diseases. Even the abovementioned traditional perception of Hahnemann's 'Law of Similar' is not sufficient enough to provide an explanation of regular

---

[73] Irvine Loudon, "A brief history of homeopathy", JSRM
https://www.ncbi.nlm.nih.gov/pmc/articles/PMC1676328/
[74] Daniel Eskinazi, "Homeopathy Re-revisited: Is Homeopathy Compatible With Biomedical Observations?" JAMA International Medicine.
https://jamanetwork.com/journals/jamainternalmedicine/fullarticle/485127
[75] Wikipedia. "Homoeopathy", https://en.wikipedia.org/wiki/Homeopathy

observations of the effects of Homoeopathic medicines. Can 'Law of Similar' explain why in a number of cases the symptoms of the patients aggravate? Is it not paradoxical to prescribe a medicine (which causes fever to a healthy person) to a patient of fever?

6
HAHNEMANN'S POSTULATION AND WARNER'S *MOMENTUM*

The counter immune response which any poisonous substance induces in human body has been manipulated by a number of different therapeutic methods such as isopathy, immunotherapy, vaccination, etc differently. The techniques and strategies of manipulating the counter immune responses make all those differences. So, if the law of "similia similibus curantur" is taken into consideration in its literal sense, isopathy and vaccination can be broadly aligned with the mainstream homoeopathic philosophy. Whereas for vaccination, dead or attenuated germs of the same disease are used to induce adaptive immunity as prophylaxis of the same disease before the infection, dead or attenuated germs of a disease are used to induce immune response against any disease after the infection. In homoeopathy, there are no rigorous criteria that the immune-response inducer must be of the same disease; rather traditionally it is believed that the medicines are selected according to the similarity of symptoms, though the 'selection of medicine according to the similarity of symptoms' is not always true. For example, check the rubrics from any homoeopathy repertory and the suggested medicines for them. You will find that almost of thirty percent of the symptoms are missing in the suggested medicines in the Materia Medica. I am doubtful whether some of those symptoms were produced during the proving of the related medicine. For example, open the "stomach" chapter of the Synthesis by Dr. Frederick Shroyens and such for the rubrics, "nausea>coition, during: Sil, Sabad", "nausea > bread after: Ant C, Zinc", "Nausea> amorous caresses, from: Ant C, Sabad", etc. I checked for the related medicines in several Materia Medicas. Unfortunately I found them missing. So, I am almost sure that selection of homoeopathic medicines is not determined by the 'law of similarity' alone. Rather evidences of successful clinical experiences have helped those medicines to make a place in the repertory.

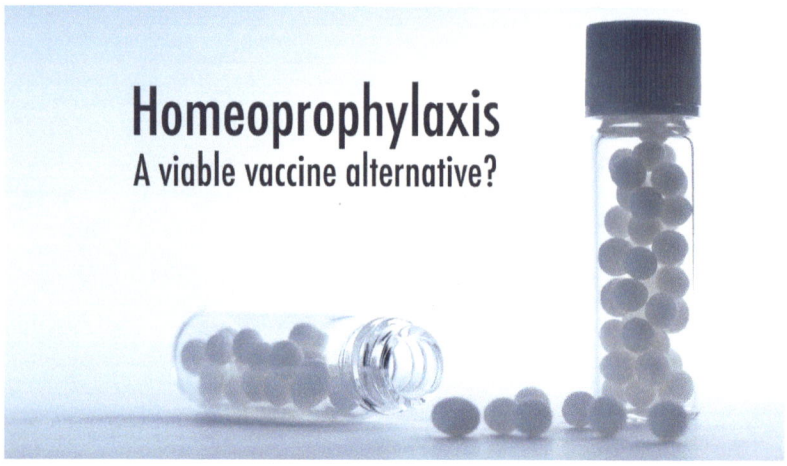

So selections of homoeopathic medicines are determined by a broad array of techniques and strategies of inducing the desired immune reactions against diseases and illness. Isopathy and vaccination fall in this broad arena of homoeopathy. Yet though Isopathy is practiced to a reasonable extent in homoeopathy, the homoeopaths are divided on acknowledging vaccinations as safe prophylaxis of diseases. Not here; I will discuss somewhere else about the business of selling the fear of the Bogus in the name of vaccination. However, I must say that the mechanism of function of vaccination is quite effective to prevent any target disease. Scholars have always stumbled on the question if it is possible to develop successful immune defense (with medicines which produce similar symptoms) against a disease which a patient already is suffering from. Let depict the situation in an example:

Suppose, a patient X is suffering from whooping cough which is caused by a type of bacteria called Bordetella pertussis.[76] According to the mechanism of vaccination, if some attenuated or dead germs of Bordetella are pushed into human body, the immune system will develop adaptive resistance against future attack of these bacteria. But if some attenuated or dead germs of pertussis are pushed into a patient of whooping cough, is it possible that those germs will induce the immune system to develop immune response which will annihilate the existing germs of Bordetella pertussis? If so, how is it possible that the immune system will develop a response (against those attenuated germs) which will be strong enough to annihilate the existing ones (we must keep it in our mind that the immune system has already failed to develop

---

[76] Mayo Clinic. "Whooping Cough". https://www.mayoclinic.org/diseases-conditions/whooping-cough/symptoms-causes/syc-20378973

immunity; otherwise the patient would not need to take the attenuated germs to get relief of suffering). Here, isopathy cannot provide any satisfactory answer. However, homoeopathic philosophy can explain if the attenuated or dead germs can cure the disease or not.

While considering the homoeopathic explanation, we must not be biased with the allopathic culture of finding out a scapegoat. Earlier I have discussed that disease according to homoeopathic philosophy is the untuned state of the *vital force* (immune system). Read what Hahnemann says in the beginning of Aphorism 29: "Any disease that is not exclusively a surgical case consists of a particular pathological, dynamic untunement of feelings and functions in our *vital force* (vital principle)"[77] So, the prime focus of homoeopathic medication is to agitate the *vital force* to get back to its earlier tuned state, not to kill Bordetella pertussis because killing the germs is, indeed, the task of the tuned *vital force*. How do Homoeopathic medicines perform this task of restoring the untuned *vital force* to the state of tuneness? In the Organon of Medicine, Hahnemann argued that an essential biological property (vital principle) of *Vital force* (immune system) can harmlessly be manipulated to bring the untuned *vital force* into the state of tuneness. Hahnemann did not use any specific term to denote this biological property or vital function. Let us name it as Hahnemann's Postulation or Warner's Postulation (why will I not associate my own name with this great man's great discovery?). Hahnemann describes it in Aphorism 29 as following:

> So in homoeopathic cure this vital principle, which has been dynamically untuned by natural disease, is taken over by a similar and somewhat stronger artificial disease, through the administration of a potentized medicine that has been accurately chosen for the similarity of its symptoms. Consequently the (weaker) natural dynamic disease is extinguished and disappears; from then on it no longer exists for the vital principle, which is controlled and occupied only by the stronger artificial disease; this in turn presently wanes, so that the patient is left free and cured.[78]

Let's decode what Hahnemann want to say about the mechanism of action of his medicine. In this aphorism, Hahnemann mentions two disease forces a. natural disease (the weaker one) which is caused by the natural *disease-agent* or outer malefic disease force, b. artificial disease which is similar and somewhat stronger artificial and caused by potentized medicines. In aphorism 18, he describes which properties a substance should have in order to be the medicine, as he says, "medicines can cure disease only if they possess the power to alter the way a person feels and functions".[79] Hence, he claims that

---

[77] Samuel Hahneman, Organon of Medicine, Para-29
[78] Samuel Hahneman, Organon of Medicine, Para-29

the vital principle is "taken over by a similar and somewhat stronger artificial disease" and subsequently, "the (weaker) natural dynamic disease is extinguished and disappears; from then on it no longer exists for the vital principle, which is controlled and occupied only by the stronger artificial disease". This explanation of Hahnemann about the mechanism of action is very much metaphoric, as Hahnemann does not have any concrete scientific proof. He reached this conclusion which he deduced rationally from his observations. So, he failed to explain why the weaker natural dynamic disease disappears and no longer exists for the vital principle. But obviously a modern immunological interpretation of Hahnemann's explanation provides a very clear scenario of why the weaker natural dynamic disease disappears and no longer exists for the vital principle. Earlier in this book, I have shown that Hahnemann's concepts such as *vital force*, vital principles, *miasm*, *disease-agent*, etc are, indeed, the philosophical predecessors of the modern immunological terminologies such as immune system, immune functions, states of immune deficiencies, pathogens, etc. However, let us propose a modern interpretation of Hahnemann's postulation:

> If the immune system (*vital force*) detects two (almost) similar threats simultaneously, the immune responses (actions of vital principles) which are metered by the severer one consider both threats as one unitary target and treat them with the same defense and recuperative strategies. During the immune responses in action, the less severe infection will be cured faster than the severer one. (Let's consider it as Hahnemann's Postulation)

Indeed, the abovementioned postulation is one of the greatest discoveries of modern biological science. Hahnemann provides many examples of such biological phenomena, as he says, "A disease of many years' duration being cured by an outbreak of smallpox or measles – both of these running that course in a few weeks – is a similar occurrence".[80] Hahnemann spent the entirety of Aphorism 46 to a number of such phenomena:

> a. Smallpox, prominent among them and so notorious forits many violent symptoms, has removed and cured a host of ills that have similar symptoms. b. A person who was blind for two years after the suppression of a scalp eruption completely recovered his sight after smallpox, according to Klein. c. A person who was blind for two years after the suppression of a scalp eruption completely recovered his sight after smallpox, according to Klein. d. A chronic herpetic eruption was cured (homeopathically) promptly, completely, and permanently by and eruption of measles.[81]

---

[79] Samuel Hahneman, Organon of Medicine, Para-18
[80] Samuel Hahneman, Organon of Medicine, Para-29

Hahnemann's painstaking research on the discovery of such biological phenomenon helped him to manipulate it therapeutically. In order to manipulate this phenomenon therapeutically, he provided some criteria for the medicine to be considered as therapeutic. First of all, the medicine must "possess the power to alter the way a person feels and functions".[82] Again, he describes the essential characteristics of homoeopathic medicines as following: "Every real medicine can at all times and in all circumstances affect every living person and bring about its particular symptoms in him (even clearly perceptible ones if the dose is large enough)."[83] This ability of the medicine to alter must be stronger than the *disease-agent*s. The immunological interpretation of such claim is as following: the medicine must be able to induce a stronger symptomatic immune response than the disease symptoms. Here one may ask: Why are the stronger medicine-induced symptomatic immune responses so necessary? Read again between the lines of Hahnemann's postulation and take a special note to the defense and the recuperative strategies which are adopted by the immune system (*vital force*). These strategies of the immune system (*vital force*) are the most important parts of the mechanism of actions of the homoeopathic medicines. While annihilating the threats of the medicines, the immune system also aims at curing the threats of natural disease.

Secondly, the artificial disease must be short-active and short-lived, as he says in the following statement from Aphorism 29: "The *vital force* frees itself much more easily from artificial diseases than from natural ones, although the former are stronger, because the *disease-agent*s called medicines producing the artificial diseases have a short action."[84] Can you believe that Hahnemann amazingly speculate the immunologic characteristics of his medicines almost correctly despite having no knowledge of the immune science? Indeed, the stronger but short-lived actions of the medicines are ensured by controlling the doses and choosing the most effective site of administration. By the first criterion, the medicinal substance is a severe poison the smallest amount of which can induce the strongest immune responses. All of these medicines are administered at the lowest doses at the most effective site of administration (please read the Chapter: the Most Effective Site of Administration). Upon administering the medicines, they induce a sharply uplifted and strong response, though it is short-lived.

Thirdly, not only the medicines must induce strong immune responses (disease symptoms), but also the symptoms they induce must be almost similar to the disease symptoms, as Hahnemann says: "the artificial disease brought on by a medicine does not have only to be stronger in order to cure

---

[81] Samuel Hahneman, Organon of Medicine, Para-46
[82] Samuel Hahneman, Organon of Medicine, Para-18
[83] Samuel Hahneman, Organon of Medicine, Para-32
[84] Samuel Hahneman, Organon of Medicine, Para-29

the natural disease. Above all it must have the greatest possible similarity to the natural disease being treated."[85] In all the aphorisms from Aphorism34 to Aphorism38, Hahnemann argued why the medicinal symptoms should be similar to the natural disease symptoms. However, he argued in his own way with the knowledge and empirical evidences which he had at hands during his era. Providing examples of affections with diseases which do not have similarities of symptoms, he concluded that "since nature itself cannot cure even a somewhat old disease by adding a new dissimilar one"[86], similarity between medicinal symptoms and disease symptoms is an essential criterion for any substance to be considered as medicine.

Here, one may ask what the scientific logics behind such claims of Hahnemann are. Why should a medicinal substance have the properties of inducing strong immune responses, short-active effects and similarity of symptoms? If you read Hahnemann's postulation again, you will clearly understand that the first property of inducing stronger immune response is aimed to pose the severer threat to the immune system (*vital force*). The essence of this property lies in evoking the immune system (*vital force*) to spring to action against the medicinal threat. Now if the medicinal dose is large, the medicinal sufferings are also higher and the attention of the threatened immune system or *vital force* is more focused on the medicinal threat itself. Because of the diverted immune focus, the cure of the target disease is delayed. So, Hahnemann developed a strategy to increase the *momentum* of the threat while reducing the dose in order to minimize medicinal harms. Let us call it "Warner's *Momentum*". Developing Warner's *Momentum* is a very much essential part of the mechanism of homoeopathic medicines. The first and foremost target of the homoeopathic medicine is to induce the desired immune responses and to manipulate the immune responses to cure the disease. The success of achieving this target depends on developing enough *momentum* of threat which compels the immune system to address all the similar threats existing in the body. When the dose is larger, the *momentum* of threat to the immune system is higher. So, the immune system is easily induced to develop immune responses by the *threat momentum* which is created by the large dose. But when the dose is small in order to avoid medicinal harms, the *threat momentum* of the dose also diminishes. But a number of techniques such as repeating the dose over a period of time, administering the medicines at the site which will induce the severest immune responses, etc can increase the *threat momentum* of a medicine despite its smallest amount or dose.

---

[85] Samuel Hahneman, Organon of Medicine, Para-34
[86] Samuel Hahneman, Organon of Medicine, Para-34

7
MECHANISM-OF-ACTION OF HOMOEOPATHIC MEDICINES AND WARNER'S *MOMENTUM*

However, what is Homoeopathy then? Nope, it is not simple prescribing of medicines which produce the same symptoms in healthy person. In the Organon of Medicine, Hahnemann has endeavored to describe the essence of Homoeopathy as a method of treatment which must not interfere or suppress the functions of the *vital force*, but stimulate the *vital force* to take initiatives against any pathogens or pathogenic conditions with inimical substances against which the *vital force* spontaneously initiates immune response. I think all the answers of the questions about Homoeopathy lie in this perception. Obviously, this definition necessarily provides a hint about how homoeopathic medicines work. Like antibiotics, Homoeopathic medicines do not kill or destroy pathogens. Neither do they interfere, like painkillers, analgesics, antihistamines, etc into biological immune-mechanisms which cause pain, fever, sufferings, etc as immune responses. Indeed, homeopathic medicines have nothing to do with the pathogens or pathogenic conditions. So, what do homoeopathic medicines do? They do nothing but being poisonous to the body. The more poisonous the substance is, the more venerated it is as a homoeopathic medicine. These poisonous substances are extremely loathed by the *vital force*. The result of such loathing is conspicuous. The immune system sprang to its feet to take immediate actions against these poisonous substances. Did Hahnemann perceive this ability of a medicinal substance to produce the same disease-symptoms as the medicine's ability to alter vital principle or medicines having equally spirit-like, dynamic effects? I think, it is so.

This is the response of the *vital force* which a homoeopath expects by heart and soul. The *vital force* troubled by the poisonous substances not only overcome the trouble created by the homoeopathic medicines, but also takes further initiatives against any similar symptoms caused by the natural pathogens. Indeed, this is the modern version of Hahnemann's explanation of how homoeopathic medicines work. The types of the immune-responses the *vital force* produces against different doses of the medicines synchronically and diachronically are to be explored in further researches. For example, a homoeopath very often uses lower power (greater dose such as 3x, 6x, 12x, etc) of Silicea if he wants to produce pus in the area of infection such as abscess, carbuncle, intrusion of foreign-body, etc. But there is a popular belief that higher power (lower dose such as 200, 1M, 10M, etc) of Silicea would absorb pus from the site of infection. Very often, homoeopaths claim that higher power (potency or lower dose) will not act as effectively as lower potency for children. They further claim that some medicines stop working if they are used for a long term. Also they claim that some ailments have been cured by some medicines (in constitutional or hereditary treatment) which normally do not produce those ailments in healthy human body. Another claim is that Higher Potency should not be used frequently. Indeed, our immunologic perception of homoeopathy can fairly explain all these observations of the homoeopaths. I will further show that the science of immunologic homoeopathy is adequately can explain why the physician should start prescribing from lower potency to higher potency (from higher dose to lower dose) and why the patient should stop allopathic medications while taking homoeopathic drugs. Before explaining how Homoeopathic medicines work and examining if the observations of the homeopaths are compatible with our immunological perceptions of Homoeopathy, we will try to extract some derivatives of the treatment method which Hahnemann advocated in the Organon of Medicine are as following:

Hypothesis -1:
Within the Avogadro Limit, different doses of Homoeopathic Medicines during different durations work as antigens which invite different immune responses to different degrees. These immune responses can easily be manipulated to cure any specific diseases.

Hypothesis -2:
The more similarity between the medicines' symptoms and the disease symptoms there is, the more the probability of producing the specific purgative response is. Similar pathogenic conditions in human body will induce/invite/provoke the immune system to take similar anti-pathogenic measures. Hence, the strongest, but quickly subsiding and easily surrendering to the immune system, pathogenic condition can have therapeutic effects on the long lasting and severer pathogenic condition by inducing the IS to respond to it effectively.

Hypothesis -3:
Probability of Interactions between the Immune-System and the pathogens are enhanced by the IS's ability to produce antibodies specific

to antigens of pathogens.

Hypothesis -4:
The more specific and multi-arrayed immune responses an immune unit can produce, the abler the Immune System is. The probability of the production of specific and effective Purgative Antibody is determined by both the toxicity of the medicines, the Immune System's ability to respond to the pathogen, to learn from its failure to defend it and to produce different sets of immune response both synchronically and diachronically.

Hypothesis -5:
Inhibiting an immune process is provoking an Immune System to adapt a pathogen or a pathogenic condition as a normal physiological function, called Immune Tolerance (TI). Long term immune failure also may lead to such immune tolerance, which may affect other immune units of the body.

Hypothesis-6:
Inhibiting an immune process is provoking an Immune System to adapt a pathogen or a pathogenic condition as a normal physiological function, called Immune Tolerance (TI). Long term immune failure also may lead to such immune tolerance, which may affect other immune units of the body.

Hypothesis-7:
An Immune System's interactions with a pathogen or a pathogenic condition most probably reveal itself through a man's psychophysical and behavioral symptoms both synchronically and diachronically. Though the physical symptoms caused by a particular pathogen are determinable, the behavioral and psychological symptoms are almost indeterminable.

Hypothesis-8:
Pathogens or pathogenic conditions, causing damages to the nervous system's guardianship in the immune function are more serious than those causing damages to body functions.

The simplest mechanism of action of homoeopathic medicines can be exemplified with the use of Silicea for the intrusion of foreign body. In order to understand the mechanism-of-action of Silicea, we will apply the intersectional binary operation of the Set Theory. Suppose a medicine T creates a set of threats to an organism. So the set T will be as following:

$$T = \{ T_a, T_b, T_c, T_d, T_e, T_f, T_g, T_h \ldots \}$$

[Ta, Tb, Tc etc are threats to organism]

Against this set of threats, the set of immune responses is TR:

TR = { Ra, Rb, Rc, Rd, Re, Rf, Rg, Rh …….. }
[Ra, Rb, Rc etc are organism's immune response against specific threats]

Suppose again, a splinter or a fishbone has got stuck in the throat/leg of a patient and there is poking pain in the injured area. For some unknown reasons, the patient's immune system is not producing enough phagocytes which are supposed to consume the splinter and to produce pus in order to throw it out. The set of splinter/fishbone's threats to the body is P:

P = { Tc, Te, Tf, Th }

Now, the immune responses against the threats { Tc, Te, Tf, Th } of P should be as following:

PR = { Rc, Re, Rf, Rh }

But we have supposed that the PR response set is absent either partially or completely. In such cases, if several doses of diluted T are administered at the oral route, the nociceptors of the neuroimmune system will immediately detect the threats posed by the molecules of T. Infuriated by the possible threats, the immune system will start the response set TR { Ra, Rb, Rc, Rd, Re, Rf, Rg, Rh …….. } against the threat set T { Ta, Tb, Tc, Td, Te, Tf, Tg, Th …….. }. Now, the threat sets T and P have some elements in common, the intersection of T and P will be:

T ∩ P
Or,   { Ta, Tb, Tc, Td, Te, Tf, Tg, Th …….. } ∩ { Tc, Te, Tf, Th }
Or,   { Tc, Te, Tf, Th }

According to Hahnemann's postulation, if the *vital force* (or immune system) encounter multiple similar threats at a time, the immune responses are determined by the severe ones and all the immune threats are addressed by the same immune responses. So, when the immune system is threatened by the molecules of T, it addresses the threats with PR response-set {Ra, Rb, Rc, Rd, Re, Rf, Rg, Rh ……..}. Since threats {Tc, Te, Tf, Th} are common in both of the threat sets, the PR response set {Ra, Rb, Rc, Rd, Re, Rf, Rg, Rh ……..} will cure the threats of the medicinal molecules along with the threats posed by the foreign body splinter.

The immune response to the lower potency of Silicea is very much similar to the immune response which a foreign body (inert) normally induces in human body. The array of immune responses which are induced by a foreign body along the duration from the intrusion to the expulsion is also induced by the different doses of Silicea. However, is it possible to theorize the dose-response relationship? Let's try. In this regard, we take the homoeopathic concept of disease into consideration again. According to the Organon of Medicine, disease is indeed the troubled state of the *vital force*. Suppose, a thin sharp and pointed metal of 1 millimeter length has intruded the muscle of your palm and caused damage a number of the cells. Here, though Orthodox school will tell you that the disease is the pain and inflammation, for the homoeopaths the disease is the disorder of the immune system (*vital force*) and the prospect of further casualties by the foreign body, whereas the pain and inflammation is the immune system's language of telling its disordered and threatened state. So, treating the pain and inflammation in an immune-suppressive (or immune-inhibitory) manner, instead of treating the man or the *vital force*, is to shut the immune system up forcefully. Even there is a significant difference between the ways how Allopathy and Homoeopathy see the foreign body as the apparent cause of the sufferings. According to Allopathic view, the foreign body is considered as a crucial cause of the sufferings. So, its removal is a crucial part of the treatment. This removal involves a long range of techniques such as surgery, use of medicines to kill and destroy the foreign bodies, etc. But this treatment method has a missing but very important part, that is the role of the immune system in the removal of the foreign body and repairing the damage. But from a homoeopathic viewpoint, the foreign body is nothing but a mere item in the to-do list which will be accomplished by the immune system. If the removal of the foreign body cannot be accomplished by the immune system, surgery is needed. So, when homoeopathy considers surgery and destruction of foreign body as an unnecessary option if the immune system is capable of expelling it, the Allopaths will unabashedly throw a patient to their Operation Theatre. However, let's see if it is possible to theorize when surgery or chemotherapy is needed in homoeopathy:

Vital Power ≈ Disease power
Or, Ability of the immune system ≈ Power of the *disease-agent*
Or, AIS ≈ PDA ....(1)

If we try to a graphical picture of the abovementioned equation, we will see that the ups and downs of the Engagement curve of *vital force*/immune system with pathogen/pathogenic conditions are determined by several factors such as psychological and physical wellbeing, lifestyle, occupation, eating habit, etc. The graphical presentation is as following:

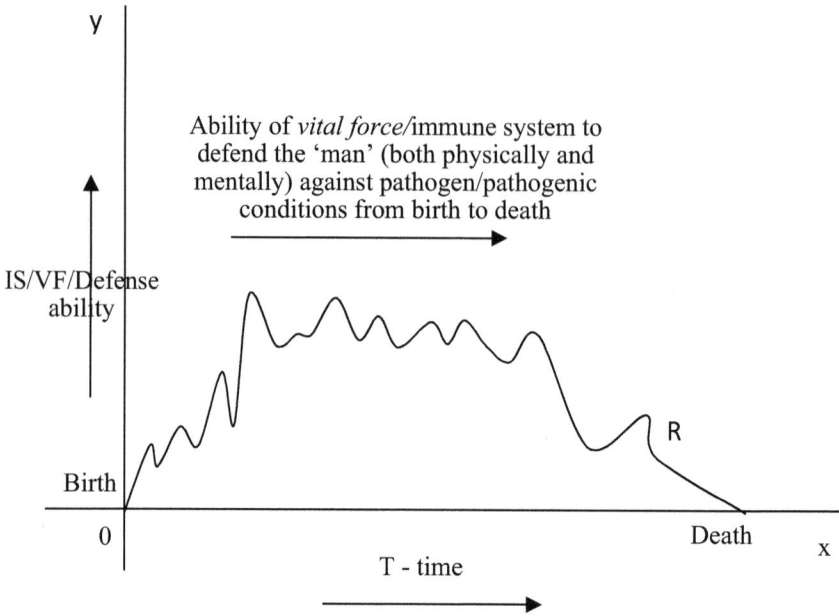

According to Hahnemann, the understanding of the balance between *vital force* and disease force is very much crucial to perceive when to resort to surgery. The abovementioned equation is too general to depict the complex relationship between the immune system (*vital force*) and the *disease-agent*; yet it can render an overall picture of the sickness of a man. In disease, the immune system is supposed to be in a losing state as following:

AIS < PDA
Or, PDA > AIS

Where,
AIS = Ability of the immune system
PDA = Power of *disease-agent*

The reversal of this balance depends on both the ability of the immune system and the power of the *disease-agent*. Whereas homoeopathy takes both sides of this equation into consideration, the allopaths are partially obsessed with the *disease-agent*s, paying no attention to the ability of the immune system. As a result, there are innumerous instances of cures of cases simply by homoeopathic medicines, where, for the allopaths, surgery was the only option. We will try to know if the abovementioned equation can help you to understand where surgery is necessary and where not. According to Hahnemann, a homoeopath's sole target is to reverse the balance between *vital force* and *disease-agent*. This sacred effort can be impeded by factors of the *vital force* and the disease. For example, the *vital force* in diseased state is directly and indirectly controlled by the following factors:

$$AIS = MS + HF + PF + CS + SM$$

Where,
AIS = Ability of the immune system
MS = *miasm* State
Hf = Hereditary Factors
PF = Psychological Factors
CS = Constitutional State
SM = Suppressive medication
C = Causation

In the similar fashion, we can sum up the factors that constitute the power of the *disease-agent* as following:

$$PDA = AEI + ASH + RFB + TFB$$

Where,
PDA = Power of *disease-agent*
AEI = Ability to evade the immune system
ASH = Ability to stay in the host
RFB = Reproducibility of the foreign bodies
TFB = Toxicity of the foreign bodies

So, if in any condition where one or more than one of the variables is such that the equation can never be reversed into AIS < PDA because the immune system is not able to get the upper hand over the disease force in the battle unless an interference in favor, surgery may be necessary. Now, we will see how the homoeopathic medicine Silicea induces immune responses to different doses along different durations. In this regard, we will know more specifically the steps which the immune system takes to clear out any foreign body from the host. Normally, for the immune system, the Silicea or Silicon Dioxide (SiO_2) is an antigen which will be ingested by macrophages which will "set off an inflammatory response by releasing tumor necrosis factors, interleukin-1, leukotriene B4 and other cytokines".[87] Wikipedia further says,

---

[87] Wikipedia. "Silicosis". https://en.wikipedia.org/wiki/Silicosis

In turn, these stimulate fibroblasts to proliferate and produce collagen around the silica particle, thus resulting in fibrosis and the formation of the nodular lesions. The inflammatory effects of crystalline silica are apparently mediated by the NALP3 inflammasome.[88]

So, each of the immune responses elicited by Silicea is very much important for a homoeopath, because his sole target is to manipulate any of them to achieve the desired result in treatment. Obviously, we must lead more researches to discover the dose-response relationship of Silicea as well as other Homoeopathic medicines. But in this book, I will simply describe the theoretical aspects of the dose-response relationship of Silicea. If we consider the abovementioned equation for Silicea as a disease force, we will get the following:

$$AIS < PDA$$
Or, $AIS < AEI + ASH + RFB + TFB$
(because $PDA = AEI + ASH + RFB + TFB$)

Where,
AIS = Ability of the immune system
PDA = Power of *disease-agent*
AEI = Ability to evade the immune system
ASH = Ability to stay in the host
RFB = Reproducibility of the foreign bodies
TFB = Toxicity of the foreign bodies

For Silicon Dioxide particles, the virulence factors AEI, ASH and RFB are almost equal to zero. So, the immune system can easily get dominance over the particles, and therefore, over TFB. However, when the balance is AIS < AEI, the immune system is in offensive mode. But when the balance is reversed into AIS > AEI, it returns to the nursing mode. In both modes, the immune system reacts differently. For a single dose of Silicea, the VF graph will be as following:

---

[88] Wikipedia. "Silicosis".

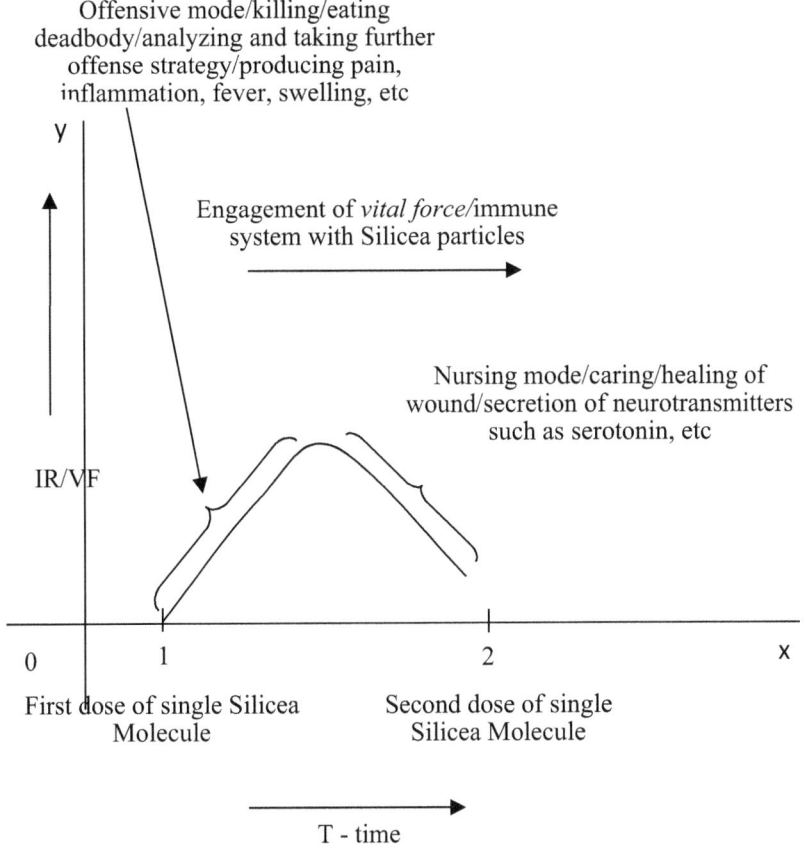

Figure: Immune Response curve for Silicea Dose

Obviously, this immune response is unitary which is made theoretically speaking against a single Silicea molecule. So, if the unitary or molecular immune response is μ, then IR or VF is:

IR (or VF) = $n\,\mu$

Where, n is the number of threatening molecules of Silicea. So, if you increase the number of Silicea particles in the dose, the response curve will expand along both X and Y axis. In the following graph, the P point on the curve indicates a stage where the immune system starts to be threatened and incapacitated by the disease force or medicinal pathogens because the immune system cannot overcome a dose which is larger than PR and because the immune system needs to have an immune response (to neutralize such a large dose), which is beyond its capacity.

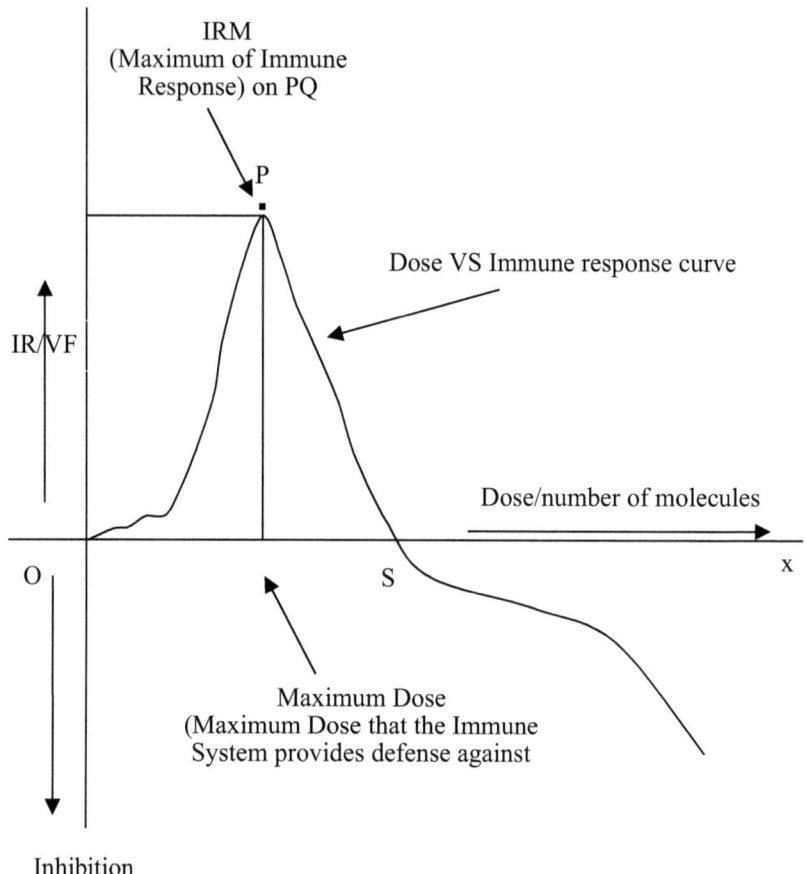

At any point on the OP slope, the immune system behaves differently against different doses. The more the dose increases (up to RP), the more violently the immune system reacts. So, when the dose increases along the OP slope, the symptoms (medicinal aggravations) of the medicinal pathogens are more and more visible towards the P end and along the PS slope, the inhibitory effect of the medicines increases along the increase of the dose. Hahnemann tells about this inhibitory effect of large dose in the following: "A medicine given in too large a dose, though completely homoeopathic to the case and in itself of a beneficial nature, will still harm the patient by its quantity and unnecessarily strong action on the *vital force*".[89] The required time which the immune system takes to overcome the dose also increases towards the end. At the same time, you must note that the stimulation of the immune system increases along the OP slope towards the P end. Hence, we need a position B which indicates the minimum dose of the medicinal antigen and the correlated highest possible stimulation of the immune system in order to avoid the medicinal aggravation.

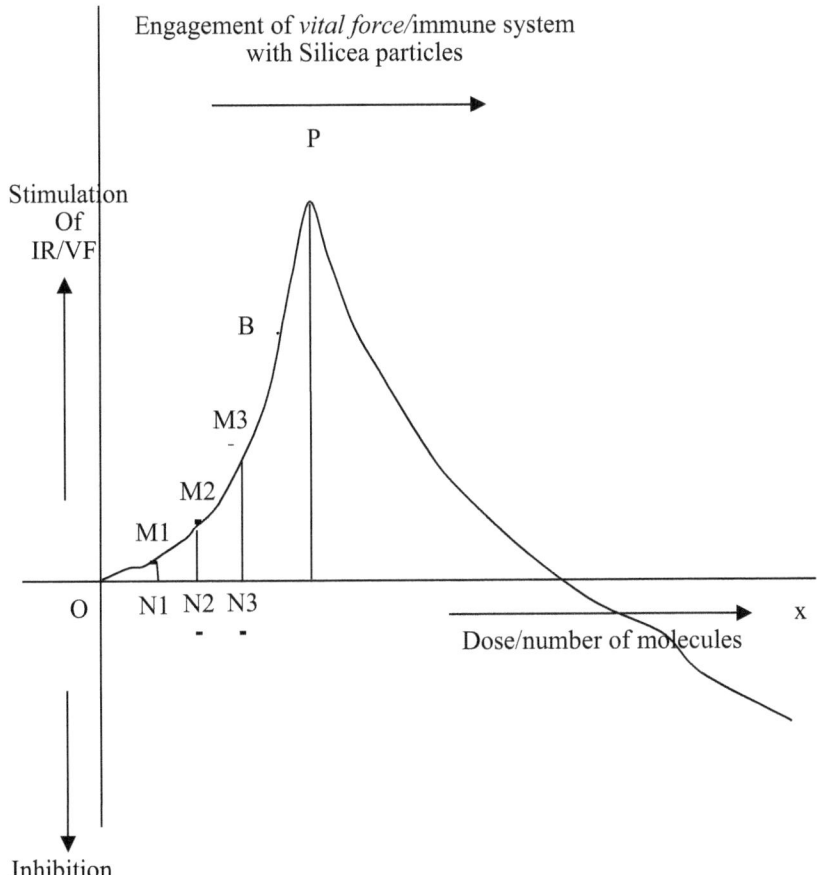

Another dilemma which a homoeopath has to deal with is to decide the

---

[89] Samuel Hahneman, Organon of Medicine, Para-275

dose which will stimulate the immune system to produce so much immune response which will be adequate enough to take initiative against the existing invasion of the external disease force. It means that the dose should be large enough to start the desired immune response and not be large so much that it starts to put extra pressure on the immune system. This claim about the quality of the dose has also been affirmed by Hahnemann in the following lines: "the dose of....homoeopathic remedy....can, as a rule, not be made so small that it is not stronger than the natural disease, that it is cannot at least partially overcome it, that it cannot at least partially extinguish it in the feelings of the vital principle, that it cannot start the process of cure".[90] If we understand how homoeopathic medicines cure we will be able to determine the effective dose for different pathogenic conditions. In this regard, we will consider the intrusion of the aforementioned tiny, thin and sharp metal into the tissue of the sole as the pathogenic condition. Even after several days of its intrusion, the immune system has not been able to clear it out. Simply it is causing a bit of stitching pain. A homoeopath will most probably prescribe Silicea to produce pus in order to clear out the foreign body. But it is apparently ironical that a homoeopath will use a different dose of Silicea to absorb pus. We will explain it in the following part. We have seen the immune response against Silicea. We will also see the nature of the immune response against the foreign body and explain how the interaction between the two types of immune responses helps the physician to achieve the goal. For the aforementioned pathogen, the immune system is taking unusually long time to produce necessary immune responses. But normally the response curve like the green one should be steeper within a narrower timeframe along the x axis. But the response curve for the pathogen is staggering over an unusually longer period. Whereas a healthy immune system will start an innate immune response within 4 hours after the intrusion, this immune system did not start innate immune response even though several days passed.

---

[90] Samuel Hahneman, Organon of Medicine, Para-279

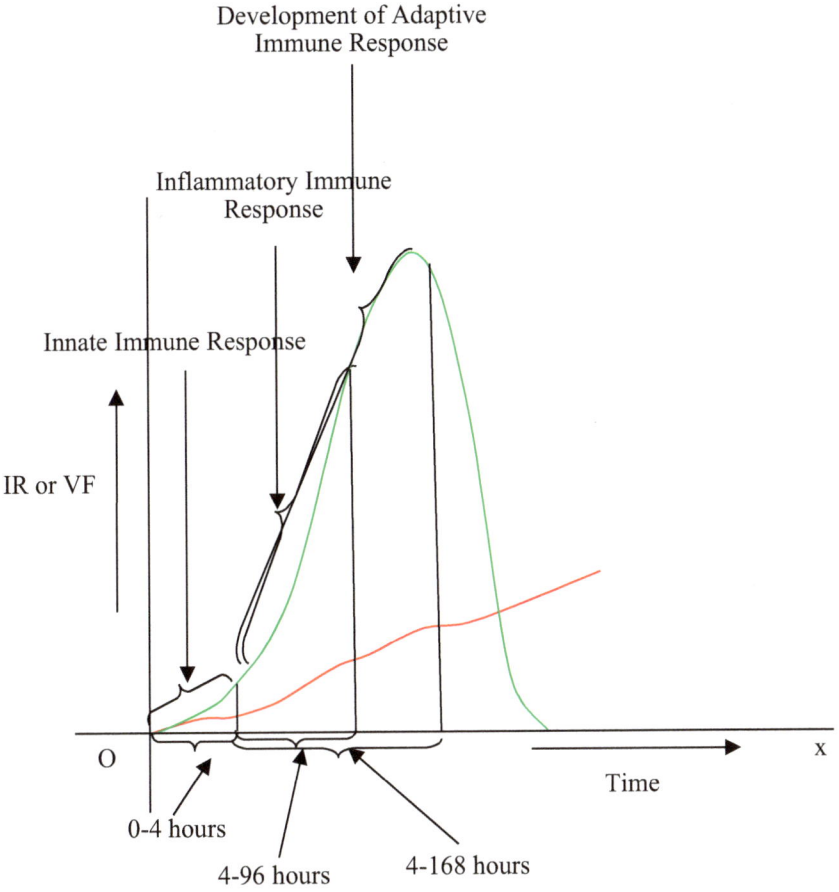

Figure 8: Response-Time Curve of Silicea

Now we will see how different doses of Silicea affect this troubled response curve (the red one). Earlier we have learnt that Silicea particles have their own response curve (the green one). As a pathogen, Silicea particles are endowed with a particular type of toxicity. So, a dose of Silicea within the medicinal limit can create a pathogenic environment which is strong enough to elicit an immune response which will be able to cover the threat caused by the foreign body. This immune response further will be divided into arrays: the first array of responses will gradually clear out the threat caused by the Silicea particles and gradually will die out. But the second array of immune responses is so much stirred and infuriated by the Silicea particles that it will be further amplified by the signal of threat caused by the foreign body. This ability to be amplified by the signal sent by the damage cells is further dependent on the threat posed by the medicinal dose, the site of administration of the drug, the immune ability, *miasm*s, psychological wellbeing and strength of the immune signal. Now we will see how different doses of Silicea affect this troubled response curve. Earlier we have learnt that Silicea particles have their own response curve. As a pathogen, Silicea particles are endowed with a particular type of toxicity. So, a dose of Silicea within the medicinal limit can create a pathogenic environment which is strong enough to elicit an immune response which will be able to cover the threat caused by the foreign body. This immune response further will be divided into arrays: the first array of responses will gradually clear out the threat caused by the Silicea particles and gradually will die out. But the second array of immune responses is so much stirred and infuriated by the Silicea particles that it will be further amplified by the signal of threat caused by the foreign body. This ability to be amplified by the signal sent by the damage cells is further dependent on the threat posed by the medicinal dose, the site of administration of the drug, the immune ability, *miasm*s, psychological wellbeing and strength of the immune signal.

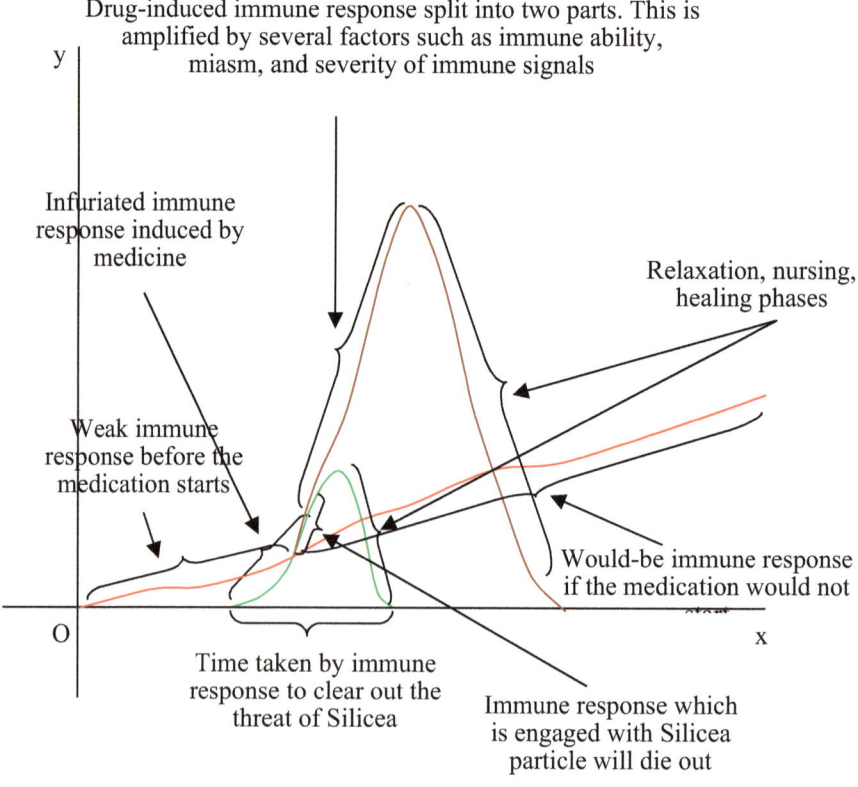

Generally, an infuriated immune system will spring to actions and address any impending threat. It will take the steps which are necessary in any particular context. For example, if the stirred immune system finds the site of injury in its initial state (the unaddressed foreign body, damaged cells, presence of cell signaling chemicals, etc), it is supposed to initiate responses which will capture the foreign body, neutralize and eat it. It will call for more help. It further will search for more threats; if there is any, it will send more specialized forces (adaptive immune responses) which will analyze the foreign body and estimate the potential threat from it. Then it will develop strategy to defend the body from future attack. Either during this whole process or at the end of the process, the immune system will adopt nursing mode. Ideally if the stirred immune system starts (provided that it is not suffering from any major drawbacks) addressing the threat, it will complete the whole cycle of its functions. So look at the "Figure: Immune Response Curve for Silicea Dose". For different Silicea doses, the curve behaves differently. Look at the following two graphs for two different doses of Silicea: Generally, an infuriated immune system will spring to actions and address any impending threat. It will take the steps which are necessary in any particular context. For example, if the stirred immune system finds the site of injury in its initial state (the unaddressed foreign body, damaged cells, presence of cell signaling chemicals, etc), it is supposed to initiate responses which will capture the foreign body, neutralize and eat it. It will call for more help. It further will search for more threats; if there is any, it will send more specialized forces (adaptive immune responses) which will analyze the foreign body and estimate the potential threat from it. Then it will develop strategy to defend the body from future attack. Either during this whole process or at the end of the process, the immune system will adopt nursing mode. Ideally if the stirred immune system starts (provided that it is not suffering from any major drawbacks) addressing the threat, it will complete the whole cycle of its functions. So look at the "Figure: Immune Response Curve for Silicea Dose". For different Silicea doses, the curve behaves differently. Look at the following two graphs for two different doses (smaller doses and larger doses) of Silicea:

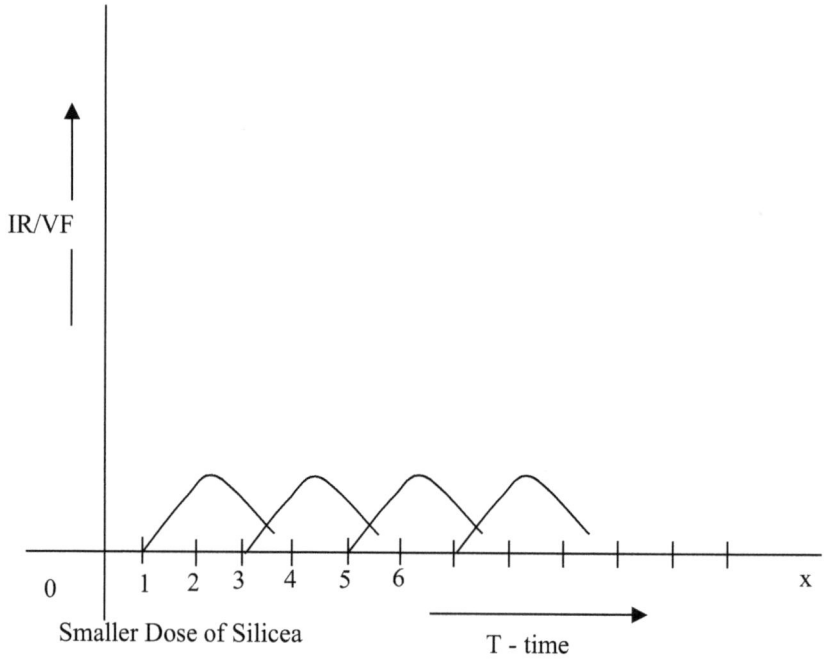

Figure: Immune response curve for repeated smaller dose

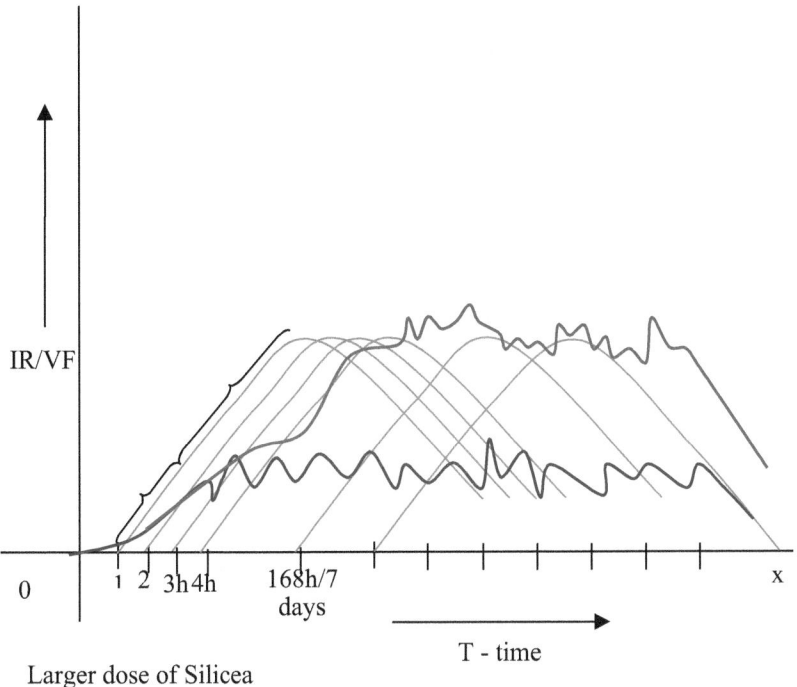

Figure: Immune Response curve for Repeated large Silicea Dose

Please note that the time covered by the response curve for the larger dose along the x axis is larger than the time taken by the response curve of the smaller dose. So, repeating the dose for a number of times will necessarily change the nature of the response curve. For example, if the successive doses occur within the innate-response period of the preceding one and if the doses are large enough not to be cleared out by innate or adaptive immune system alone, both innate and adaptive responses will remain active. In the above mentioned figure, the Green curve indicates the adaptive immune response, while the blue one refers to the innate response. So though larger doses can easily develop offensive immune responses, nursing/caring responses are continuously postponed by them because they remain busy with the offenses. On the contrary, smaller doses complete the whole phase of infection and cure within a shorter timeframe. During the infection phase, the immune responses are instigated, while during this nursing mode, the nervous system releases some neurotransmitters such Dopamine, serotonin, oxytocin, endorphins, and many others which create the feelings of happiness and wellbeing. So, smaller doses or higher potencies can bring the mental wellbeing prior to the physical cure than the larger doses or lower potencies can do. This finding is quite compatible with Hahnemann's observation:

> The signs of improvement in the emotions and mind can be expected immediately after the medicine has been taken only if the dose was small enough (i.e., as small as possible) an unnecessarily larger dose even of the most homeopathically appropriate remedy, apart from its other ill effects, acts too violently and initially disturbs the mind and emotions too strongly and too long for the patient's improvement to be noticed immediately.[91]

In order to elicit adaptive immune response the dose must be large enough to fail the innate immune response. It is because the failure of the innate immune response to clear out the threat evokes the adaptive immune response to develop. So if a man comes to a homoeopath to clear out a foreign body, the homoeopath should prescribe the larger doses. But suppose the same patient revisits the doctor with an infection where there is enough suppuration, white clammy discharge, etc. These symptoms are indicative of that the immune system has already reached the adaptive immune phase which is, for some reasons, failing to finish the task of healing the infection. In order for achieving this object of stimulating the adaptive immune response, we need a dose which can complete the whole response phase within a very short time. So, the dose must be repeated during the span from the start of adaptive immune response to the end of nursing mode. Here, the homoeopaths must keep it in their mind that since smaller doses cannot elicit adaptive immune response, it is necessary to initiate the adaptive immunity with larger doses. This strategy should be taken if the patient never took the medicine earlier. May be, gradually reducing the dose may help in this regard:

---

[91] Samuel Hahneman, Organon of Medicine, Para-253

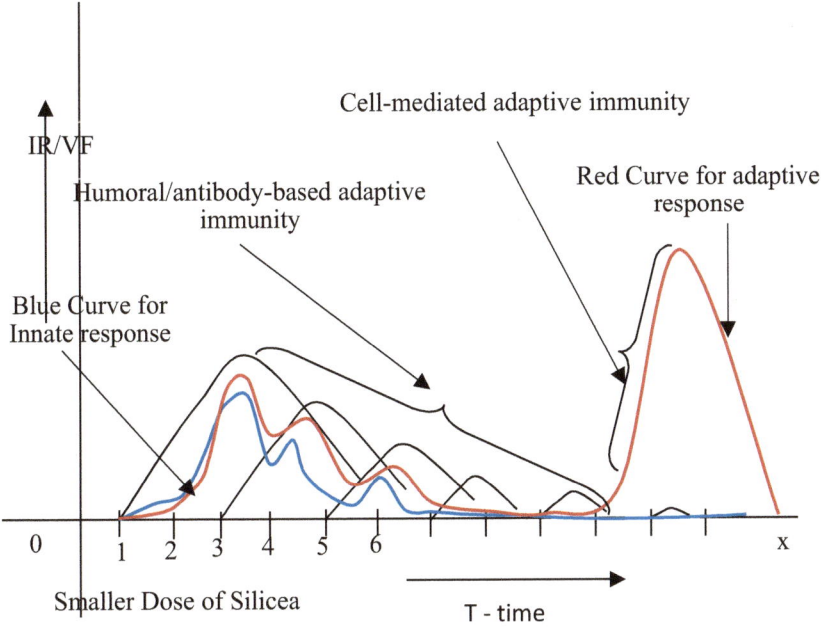

Since secondary cell-mediated immune response is specific and, therefore strong, the doses up to a certain amount seem to manifest no visual effects on the symptoms of a disease. Ask any experienced homoeopath; he/she will say that larger doses (lower potency) often do not seem to work after the administration of lower doses (higher potency). Also the homoeopaths very often face a situation that a medicine worked very well for several days, now it is not working at all. Explanation of such events is quite obvious. After a certain period of the administration of any homoeopathic medicine, the immune system develops the adaptive immune response against the medicinal particles. The adaptive immune system is quicker, more specific and more effective. It can handle larger doses up to a certain limit. So, the same dose which once worked very well to induce innate response is not working anymore now. In this situation, any large dose which is beyond the capacity of the adaptive immunity and larger than the dose which would once easily induce innate response, is supposed to induce the innate response again. The locked dose (which is quickly addressed by the adaptive immunity) fails to induce any stimulatory environment, because the repetition of the same dose at equal interval cannot create a chaotic and alarming environment which the repetition of the different dose at different intervals can create. Since increasing the dose puts an extra pressure on the immune system, this target of creating chaotic and alarming environment (which is supposed to induce immune responses and which the locked dose is now failing to create the chaotic and alarming environment) can also be achieved by decreasing the doses at a regular basis. In general an adaptive immune response on any exposure after the second one is equal to what it is for the preceding one. So, frequent recurrence of descending doses poses a fake severity of the invasion or the infection against which the immune system takes the alertest stance. Moreover, the descending doses gradually decrease the immune system's engagement with the medicinal particles and increase the amount of lymphocytes and other necessary defensive-nursing functionalities in the host. This environment is strong enough to address the infection which our patient is suffering from.

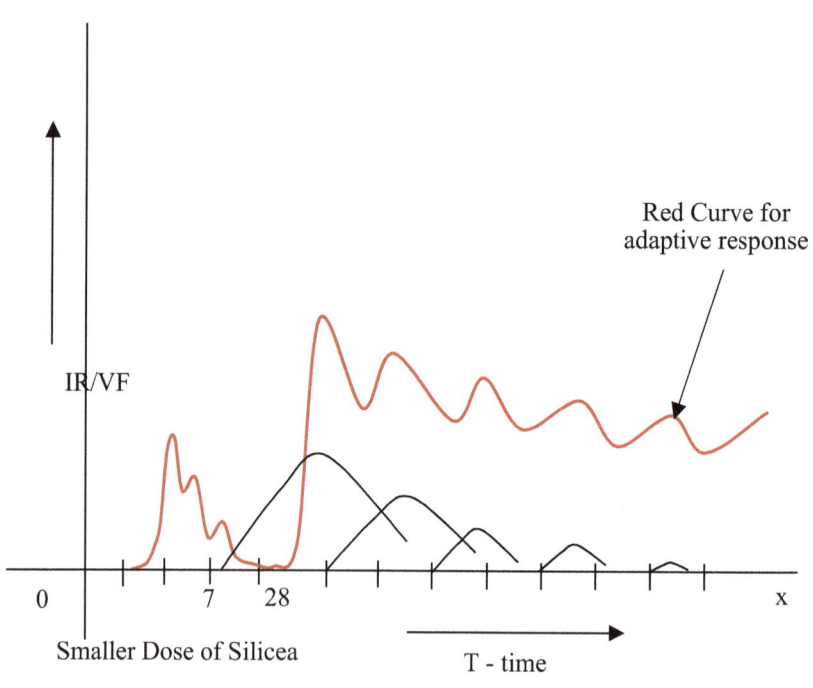

8
EFFECTIVE SITES OF ADMINISTRATION OF HOMOEOPATHIC MEDICINES

The earlier explanation of the mechanism-of-action of Silicea is one of the simplest examples of how homoeopathy medicines work. Most of the homoeopathic medicines work according to the explained way. Yet the medicines differ from one another in terms of ability to induce immune responses, types of responses they induce, the agility of responses, the duration of response, the miasms they are influenced with, types of cells they cause damages to, types of damages they cause, the sites of administration they work at the most, etc. An effective site should be the one where the lowest dose of medicinal particles stimulates the immune system the most. Obviously, a dose of medicinal particles will receive quicker and stronger immune reactions in a highly immune area than what it receives in a low immune area. In this regard, a sound knowledge of Neuroimmune system can be helpful to perceive what the most effective site of drug-administration is. The nervous system plays a very important role in the development of immune responses. The initiation of the immune response is intensively determined and controlled by the Central Nervous System (CNS). Almost all the immune organs are intimately connected with the CNS through Peripheral Nervous System (PNS). Look at what Dantzer and Wollman tell about the relationship in their article:

> The concept that the brain can modulate activity the immune system stems from the theory of stress. Recent advances in the study of the inter-relationships between the central nervous system and the immune system have demonstrated a vast network of communication pathways between the two systems.[92]

They further explained how the lymphoid organs are connected with the autonomic nervous system and how the immune functions are regulated by the membrane receptors which bind to the neurotransmitters and neuropeptides. Immune functions such as cell proliferation, chimiotactics, specific immune responses and many other vital ones are activated and regulated by the integrated neuroendocrine-immune network. In an article, "Relationships between the brain and the immune system", Dantzer and Wollman further narrate:

> The communication pathways that link the brain to the immune system are normally activated by signals from the immune system, and they serve to regulate immune responses. These signals originate from accessory immune cells such as monocytes and macrophages and they are represented mainly by proinflammatory cytokines. Proinflammatory cytokines produced at the periphery act on the brain via two major pathways: (1) a humoral pathway allowing pathogen specific molecular patterns to act on Toll-like receptors in those brain areas that are devoid of a functional blood-brain barrier, the so-called circumventricular areas; (2) a neural pathway, represented by the afferent nerves that innervate the bodily site of infection and injury. In both cases, peripherally produced cytokines induce the expression of brain cytokines that are produced by resident macrophages and microglial cells. These locally produced cytokines diffuse throughout the brain parenchyma to act on target brain areas so as to organise the central components of the host response to infection (fever, neuroendocrine activation, and sickness behavior).[93]

It is very much clear from the progress of modern researches on the role of brain in the initiation of the immune response against any foreign body that the distance between the CNS and the site of infection plays a crucial role in the quality of the immune response. The nearer the site of infection is to the CNS, the stronger the response is. Furthermore, the nearer the site of infection is to the CNS, the shorter the time which the immune system takes to develop is. Almost all the organs which are involved in the remote regulation of necessary biological and immunological functions of distant target organs through the neuroendocrine signaling system are located in or nearer to the CNS. Scientists believe that the hypothalamus plays as the neural control center for all endocrine systems, whereas the thalamus has "several functions such as relaying of sensory signals, including motor signals to the

---

[92] Dantzer R, Wollman EE. "Relationships between the brain and the immune system". J Soc Biol. 2003;197(2):81-8 in NCBI
https://www.ncbi.nlm.nih.gov/pubmed/12910622
[93] Dantzer R, Wollman EE. "Relationships between the brain and the immune system". J Soc Biol. 2003

cerebral cortex, and the regulation of consciousness, sleep, and alertness".[94] Obviously the time and the intensity of the response to any infection are related to the distance of the CNS from the site of infection. So, the theorization is quite obvious as following:

IIR α DSOI
Or, IIR = m/DSOI

Where,
IIR = Intensity of immune response
DSOI = Distance of the site of infection from the CNS

Intensity of immune response is inversely related to the distance of the site of infection from the CNS. In the similar fashion, the time which is taken by the immune system to develop against any infection is also inversely related to this distance as following:

TIR α DSOI
Or, TIR = m/DSOI

Where,
TIR = Time of immune response
DSOI = Distance of the site of infection from the CNS

The Central Nervous System plays an significant role in the immune system. So the distance between the CNS and the site of infection or site of administration is important for a number of reasons. Firstly, the hypothalamus being instigated by a number of cytokines, such as IL-1, IL-6, IL-10 and TNF-alpha takes steps to modulate the immune response through the hypothalamic–pituitary–adrenal axis (HPA axis or HTPA axis). It "regulates the immune system through neuroendocrine pathways, such as the HPA axis [which] is responsible for modulating inflammatory responses that occur throughout the body".[95] Look at the process of the pain-modulating function of the HPA axis. Proinflammatory cytokines which released into the peripheral circulation system travel through the blood brain barrier and interacts with CNS. As a result, the adrenal gland releases neurotransmitters and glucocorticoids such as cortisol, into the blood, which in turn "suppresses immune response by inhibiting the expression of proinflammatory cytokines (e.g. IL-1, TNF alpha, and IFN gamma) and increasing the levels of anti-inflammatory cytokines (e.g. IL-4, IL-10, and IL-13) in immune cells, such as

---

[94] Wikipedia. "Thalamus". https://en.wikipedia.org/wiki/Thalamus
[95] Wikipedia. "Hypothalamic–pituitary–adrenal axis". https://en.wikipedia.org/wiki/Hypothalamic–pituitary–adrenal_axis

monocytes and neutrophils".[96] So, the distance which the proinflammatory and anti-inflammatory cytokines travel through to reach the Hypothalamus and the pituitary gland plays a crucial role in determining the quality and intensity of the immune response.

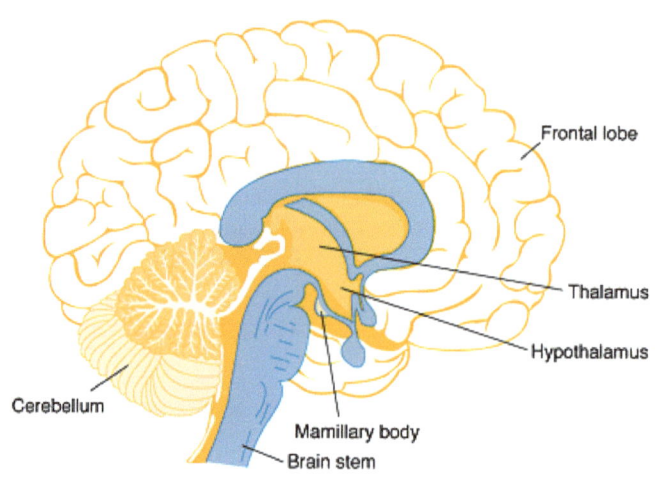

Secondly, the distance between the site of medicine-administration and the CNS is important because the sensory nervous receptor, namely nociceptor, which is responsible for "responding to potentially damaging stimuli" by sending signals to the CNS through the spinal cord to the brain needs to be close to the thalamus as well as the CNS in order to get quicker and more effective immune responses. Nociception, the process of perceiving the damaging stimuli or actual damage is one of the crucial steps in the development of immune response against any potential damage. Here, I cannot but mention a part of Aphorism 16 which clearly shows that despite having no knowledge of modern nervous system and neuroimmune science, Hahnemann could imagine the role of the neuro-receptors in perceiving the threats (for Hahnemann, it is "spirit-like, dynamic effects") of medicinal molecules, as he says, "The physician can remove these pathological untunements (diseases) only by acting on our spirit-like *vital force* with medicines having equally spirit-like, dynamic effects that are perceived by the nervous sensitivity everywhere present in the organism."[97] Read between the

---

[96] Wikipedia. "Hypothalamic–pituitary–adrenal axis"
[97] Samuel Hahneman, Organon of Medicine, Para-16

lines of any article on the Sensory Nervous System. You feel how much correct Hahnemann's assumption about the nociceptive receptors' ability to detect equally spirit-like, dynamic of medicine was. The effective development of the immune defense against any infection or damaging stimuli crucially depends on the successful transmission of the chemical messages to the brain. If the transmission of the casualty is successful, the brain receives it as some unpleasant feelings such as pain, inflammation, etc. Being provoked by the pain-message, the brain (the CNS) takes further defensive initiatives against the injury through an Integrated Network of Organs Regulatory System (INORS).

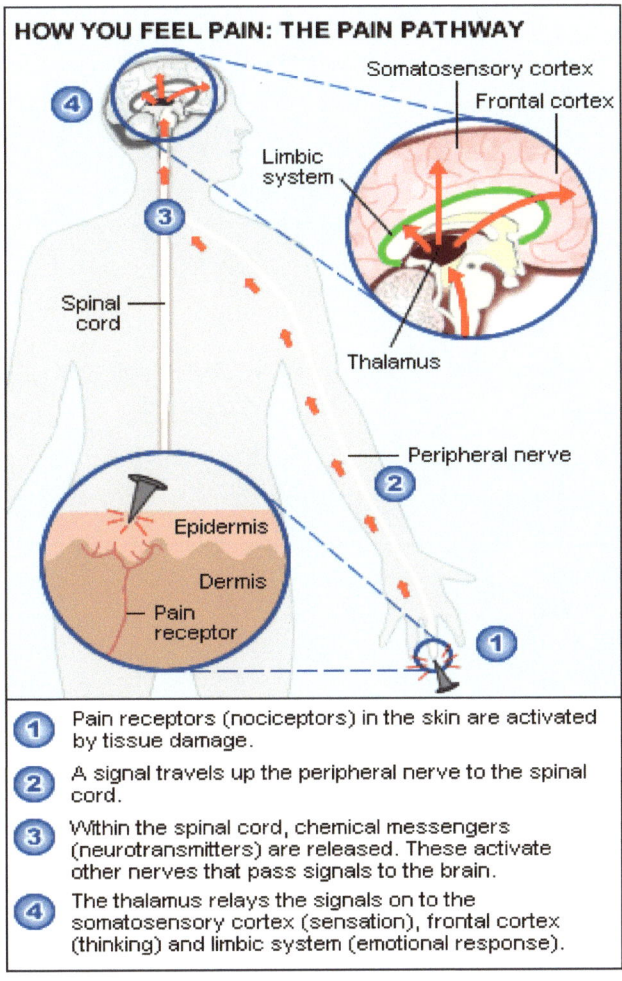

Obviously, a sound knowledge of the nerve conduction science can help us perceive about the most effective site of administration of homoeopathic medicines. In homoeopathy, the most precious property of a medicine is the immune response which it provokes the immune system to initiate. A medicine is considered as the most effective, if it is capable of inducing the most intensive immune with the least possible amount of its substance within the shortest possible timeframe, as Hahnemann says in Aphorism 18: "medicines can cure disease only if they possess the power to alter the way a person feels and functions".[98] But the distance between the CNS and the site administration also plays a crucial role in inducing the desire immune response. The signal of damaging stimuli travels all the way to the brain through different nerve at certain speeds as following. So, it is very much reasonable to assume that the site which will supposedly induce the most effective immune response is the nearest to the CNS.

Features of different types of nerve fibre

Nerve fibre	A-alpha	A-beta	A-delta	C
Appearance				
Information carried	• Position • Spatial awareness	• Touch	• Sharp pain ('fast pain') • Temperature	• Dull pain ('slow pain') • Temperature • Itch
Diameter (micrometers)	13-20	6-12	1-5	0.2-1.5
Speed of signal conduction (meters/second)	80-120	35-75	5-35	0.5-2.0

According to this distance relativity of the effectiveness of the immune response, the oral and the nasal cavities are the most effective sites of administration. Moreover, being the only two gateways which are used to get supply from external world, the oral and nasal cavities are believed to be

---

[98] Samuel Hahneman, Organon of Medicine, Para-18

highly fortified with innumerous nociceptors that are always alert against any trespasses of harmful chemicals and microorganisms. Nociceptors are supposed to "detect signals from damaged tissue or the threat of damage and indirectly also respond to chemicals released from the damaged tissue".[99] The TRP channels of the chemical nociceptors within the oral and the nasal cavities can detect a wide range of chemical stimulants such as capsaicin, acrolein, external toxins, ligands, certain fatty acid ligands, etc. Even if the damaging stimuli do not exceed the pain threshold, the immune system continues the detection and defending the noxious chemical molecules.

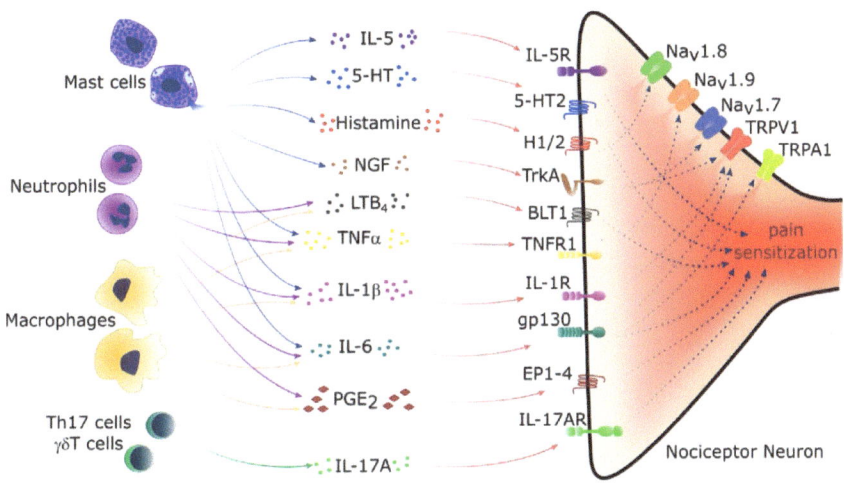

(Source: https://www.ncbi.nlm.nih.gov/pmc/articles/PMC5205568/)

Since homoeopathic medicines produce different symptoms during the proving, it will not be irrational to think that the damaging effects of the molecules of homoeopathic medicines are quickly detected by the nociceptive system of the sensory nervous system. So the scholars who wonder how it is possible for the negligible number of molecules of medicine to bring so great changes are indeed driven by some bestial impulse of filling their patients' belly with medicinal syrups. But homeopathy is free of such idiocy. Hahnemann might not have any knowledge of the noniceptive process of the sensory nervous system. But he was quite aware that the smallest doses of the

---

[99] Nachum Dafny. "Chapter 6: Pain Principles", Neuroscience Online. https://nba.uth.tmc.edu/neuroscience/m/s2/chapter06.html

poisonous molecules will be detected by the immune system (*vital force*). So he wanted to keep the subtle counter immune response (vital response) which is evoked by the subtle dose of the medicine uncorrupted and uncontaminated; as usually he advocated that: "Considering the smallness of the dose....everything that could have any medicinal action must be removed from the diet and the daily regimen, so that the subtle dose is not overwhelmed and extinguished, not even disturbed, by any foreign medicinal influence"[100] However, from the abovementioned discussion, it can further be claimed that infection or administration of homoeopathic medicine on any innervated organ initiate immune responses are stronger than those which are produced by infection or administration of medicine on any paralyzed organs. Thirdly and finally, the site of administration in a highly immune or defense area will necessarily evoke the most effective and intensive immune response. The whole immune system maintains a complex and highly sophisticated defense mechanism. It defends the organs with priority basis according to their importance and vulnerability. Traditionally it is supposed that organs within the thoracic cage and the upper organs of the body are the most important ones. So, these organs are supposed to be highly immune. Take a look at the positions of the immune organs in the following picture. Almost all of the immune organs such as tonsil, adenoid, lympathic duct and lymph nodes, are positioned above the thoracic duct. Another reason behind such defense structure of the immune organs is that they are to defend the oral and the nasal cavities in order for sterilizing the only permitted routes of intakes of external substances. So, the defense system needs to stay alert and to focus its defense effort on preventing any harmful intrusion. The immune system intimately interacts with the nervous system to keep these areas safe. Being the nearest to the Central Nervous System and the brain, the immune system can efficiently grow an interactive and communicative defense against any external harmful stimuli or substances.

Furthermore, almost all of the organs or glands which directly or indirectly regulate remote target organs in order for maintaining a healthy state are located in the brain. Functions such as maintaining core temperature through thermoregulation, blood glucose regulation, human iron metabiolism, blood-gas regulation, blood-oxygen levels, Baroreflex and Renin–angiotensin system, maintaining sodium, potassium and calcium levels, maintianance of the neuroendocrine functions through H-P-A axis and many other are directly regulated by the CNS. Any slightest intrusion (or infection) of any harmful external stimuli at the oral and the nasal cavities can easily induce immune responses and affect these functions within the shortest possible time. For example, if administered intravenously at the hand or leg, any amount of toxic substance which is far less than the pain threshold may not be capable of exerting any effects on the nerve. But the same amount will induce a

---

[100] Samuel Hahneman, Organon of Medicine, Para-259

noticeable effect on the nervous system as well as the homoeostatic functions of the body. Indeed, the effective site of administration should be the one which helps the lowest dose of MA most effectively to affect the immune system and to produce the expected purgatory antibody. According to this assessment, oral and nasal cavities are supposed to be the perfect sites of administration of homoeopathic medicines.

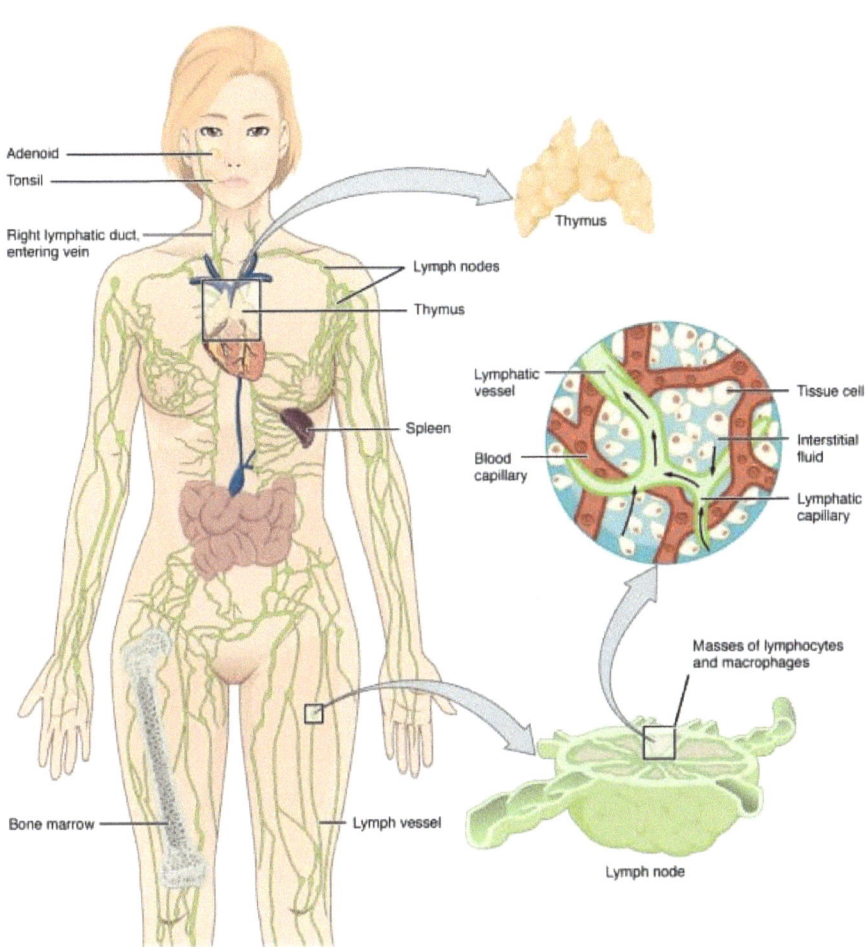

9
OUTLINE OF A HOMOEOPATHIC MATERIA MEDICA: HOW WE SHOULD READ MEDICINES?

In this chapter, I must beg your pardon. Using bombastic language is a common practice among the homeopathic authors who are from non-medical sector. No matter how much bombastic the titles of their treatment methods are! If it cannot stand off the oncoming scientific refutations, it is more than a mortal blow on Homeopathy. No other criticism from the allopathic sectors is proved to be as lethal as the adverse effects of these bombastic methods on homoeopathy are. In this book, I will not mention these methods by their name. But I will try to challenge and refute the validities of these methods. See what one of these authors is telling in the following lines:

> We prescribe on symptoms of the mind alone. This is a direct application of the principle that the health and disease of man proceeds from the centre and therefore cure must begin there also.[101]

Prescribing on mental and emotional symptom alone can be this author's monopoly. But can it be considered as a universal practice? The author made such comment without gauging how much his statement is compatible with modern biological discoveries. When he comments that "the health and disease of man proceeds from the centre", it shows that he has already failed to internalize Hahnemann's philosophy. Homoeopathic philosophy has essentially two basic aspects: the first one is purely philosophical and the second one is practical and compatible with objective reality. Failing to perceive Hahnemann's philosophy in the context of biological realities has pushed these authors to resort to mental part which is one (not only) of the most important criterion of homoeopathic treatment. Moreover, their

---

[101] Yogesh Shegal, "Revolutionized Homeopathy: Sehgal Method of Homoeopathy by Mind". https://www.homeopathy360.com/2018/02/24/revolutionized-homeopathy-sehgal-method-of-homoeopathy-by-mind/

decision to rely on the mental symptoms only and intensively has been inspired by the edibility of such mental symptoms. But who will tell them that mind (also rationality, feelings, sensations, etc) is only a part, not the whole of human existence. Moreover, who told them that mind is at the center of human existence and that the health and disease of man proceeds from the centre (mind)? Can you quote a single sentence from the Organon of Medicine which shows that disease starts from the mind alone? There is a gross failure on the authors' part to perceive the whole picture of homoeopathic pathology. In his book, Hahnemann has unequivocally used the term, '*vital force*' to denote an entity which fights for the human existence against pathogenic forces. He further asserts that disease is caused by the *vital force* when it is untuned by a number of pathogenic forces. Earlier I showed how the *vital force* causes disease. The progress of disease is quite clear. First, the body is infected by the external pathogenic forces. The *vital force* which is in control of the body is informed about the infection by some vital functions or vital principles. In response to these warning messages about the infection, some other vital functions (or vital principles) cause the emotional turmoil, emotional outbursts, tears, mental and physical pains, restlessness, fear of death, etc. Please take a look at the sequence of the steps of the progression of the disease:

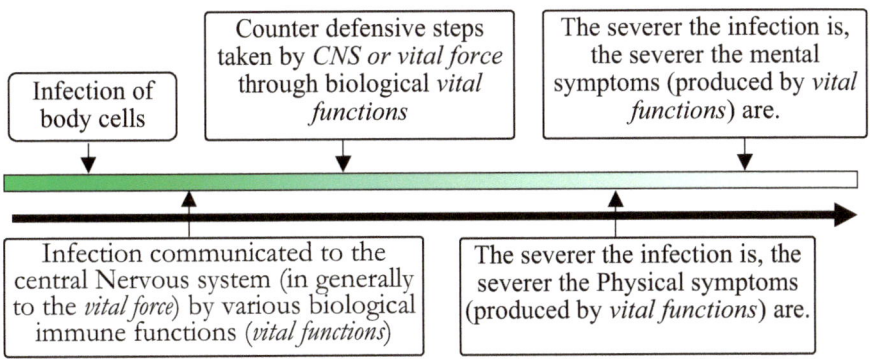

Where does the disease proceed from? Is it mind? Or is it the body? The above figure shows that it starts from body and reveals both physical and mental symptoms. In another aphorism, Hahnemann speaks of an opposite scenario. In this scenario, the *vital force* may be overstrained by mental factors such as mental overexertion, continuing emotional stress, prolonged grief and anger, etc. In such case, the disease proceeds from the mind (yet it happens mostly in chronic cases), as Hahnemann says, "The more the vital principle has been run down by debilitating passions, grief, and worry, and especially by unsuitable medical treatment, the more quickly it develops and the graver it is."[102] So, Hahnemann considered that the *vital force* can be affected principally by two types of threats: a. mental threat, exertion, turmoil, etc and b. emotional threat, exertion, stresses, etc. and these two types of threats are derived from different factors such as "the evident physical constitution of the patient, his affective and intellectual character, his activities, his way of life, his habits, his social position, his family relationships, his age, his sexual life, etc".[103] He further mentioned such factors in the Aphorism 77: "the habitual indulgence in harmful food or drink; all kinds of excesses that undermine health; prolonged deprivation of things necessary to life; unhealthy places, especially swampy regions; dwelling only in cellars, damp workplaces, or other closed quarters; lack of exercise of fresh air; physical or mental overexertion; continuing emotional stress; etc".[104] In the Organon of Medicine, Hahnemann advised in many places to uplift the impediments which may put the *vital force* under debilitating strains as following:

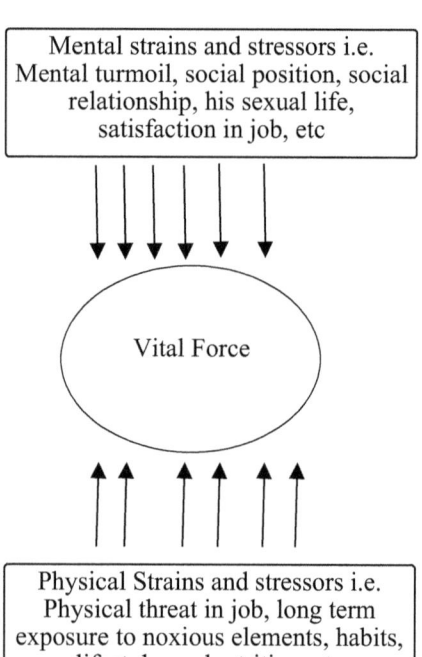

---

[102] Hahnemann, the Organon of Medicine. Aphorism 78
[103] Hahnemann, the Organon of Medicine. Aphorism 5
[104] Hahnemann, the Organon of Medicine. Aphorism 77

Hahnemann suggests that a physician's first and foremost duty is to shiver the influence of both of these mental and physical pathogenic factors. Then he or she must focus his/her attentions to restore the untuned *vital force* to its earlier tuned state with the help medicines. When there is no significant physical damage, the psychoactive properties of medicines can easily normalize the disordered psychological state. We can expect that the tuned mental state provides the *vital force* with some facilities which the *vital force* enjoys during the healthy mental state and the *vital force* without the mental stress will be able to easily address some diseases which the *vital force* with healthy mental state could cure without the help of medicines. But what about those diseases which the *vital force* could not cure on its own, even if it had been accompanied by a healthy mental state? It is clear that restoration of mental health alone cannot assist the untuned *vital force* (immune system) to roll back to its earlier tuned state. So despite the clear evidence that mind in homoeopathic pathology occupies an important but partial role, how is it possible for us to claim that disease can be cured on mind symptoms alone? What type of nonsensical mockery is it to prescribe Arsenic 30/Aconite 30 (or other medicines which are suitable for panic, fear of death and restlessness) to a child with a fishbone stuck in the throat because s/he is panicked, restless and afraid of dying (s/he thinks that the fishbone may kill him/her)? Obviously these psychoactive medicines can normalize the irritated mental state of the child. But how is it possible that these two medicines will provoke the immune system or *vital force* to expel the fishbone? We have a number of great medicines such as Silicea, Heper Sulp, Merc Sol, etc which are specialized to provoke the immune systems to produce phagocytes to gather around the fishbone and expel it. So, 'prescribing on mental symptoms alone' while ignoring the physical symptoms fairly indicates our failure to perceive the scientific essence of the homoeopathic therapeutic system. Indeed, such practice also literally opposes what Hahnemann advises in the following:

> The unprejudiced observer realizes the futility of metaphysical speculations that cannot be verified by experiment, and no matter how clever he is, he sees in any given case of disease only the disturbances of body and soul which are perceptible to the senses: subjective symptoms, incidental symptoms, objective symptoms, i.e., deviations from the former healthy condition of the individual now sick which the patient personally feels which people around him notice, which the physician sees in him.[105]

Hahnemann's pathology is nothing extraordinary; it is nothing spiritual, supernatural and metaphysical. It is almost compatible with modern pathology. Hahnemann lacks the knowledge of germs because it was discovered after his death. Yet he filled up this lack with almost similar terms,

---

[105] Hahnemann, the Organon of Medicine. Aphorism 6

"*Disease-agent*", "external factors", "intrinsic factors", etc. For Hahnemann, soul and body are meaningless without each other. Without body, soul is beyond explanation and without soul, body is lifeless. But currently there is a trend among the homoeopaths to solely depend on the mind or soul; it is nothing but their attempt to hide their failure to perceive the complex physical realities. Throughout his whole life, Hahnemann loathed any metaphysical speculation about the therapeutic methods which existed in his contemporary medical sector, as he asserts that "the unprejudiced observer realizes the futility of metaphysical speculations that cannot be verified by experiment".[106] See how some of his overenthusiastic followers like Rajan Sankaran have taken Homoeopathy to a metaphysical height from where you will never recognize the subtle but important physical realities like immune system (*vital force*), immune functions (vital functions, vital principles), nervous system, etc:

> The Sensation Approach is based on the premise that deep inside each individual, is a specific and distinct energy that shapes who we are – our likes and dislikes, the way we think, act and feel, and finally our illnesses. This energy pattern is called 'the other song'.[107]

What energy pattern is Rajan Sankaran talking of? Does it have any biological implication? Can it be proved in the laboratory? Is it, in any way, equivalent to Hahnemann's *vital force*? These authors are making Homoeopathy the laughingstock to the skeptics. Homoeopathic treatment process is based on a rich philosophy. Certainly this philosophy of Hahnemann has a lot of biological implications. But failing to understand those biological implications, these over-enthusiasts have taken the homoeopathic philosophy to an unreachable metaphysical level. Such failure provoked Yogesh Shegal to make such a pathetic claim: "We prescribe on mental symptom alone". Homoeopathic case-taking system is well-reasoned and scientific; it is quite painstaking but fitting with the aim of a physician. Very cautiously, Hahnemann has noted down the duties of a physician throughout the Organon of Medicine. A physician's duty involves painstaking scrutiny of causes of the disease (causa occasionalis), constitution of the patient, determining the miasma, discovering the patient's past and his family history and many other minute-details about the patient and the patient's surroundings. Should you prescribe on mental symptoms alone skipping all these painstaking tasks of case-taking? A patient who is suffering from whooping cough has come to your chamber and, with a breathless voice interrupted by frequent gushes of coughs, implored "Doctor! Please save my job! Save me and my family! Tomorrow I have to attend a presentation in my

---

[106] Hahnemann, the Organon of Medicine. Aphorism 6
[107] Rajan Sankaran, http://www.theothersong.com/international/sensation-method-in-homoeopathy/

office. If it continues, we will lose the 4 billion dollar contract but my cough is killing me! Give me the strong medicines so that I do not have to come again. Your chamber is far away from my house. The journey cost to your chamber is too much." Now, being inspired by the Revolutionized Homoeopathy of Dr. Yogesh Segal you will prescribe Opium 30 on the basis of the following rubrics:

- ☐ Fear, extravagance of
- ☐ Business, talks of

Imagine the scenario of the patient's second visit to your chamber again and he was telling, "I begged you to give me the most powerful medicines. Your medicines did nothing that time. I simply threw the money just into water. I had to take Antitussive before the presentation for my UK buyers. The seminar presentation was very crucial for my business. Please this time give me the effective medicines. Again I have to attend another one. But this cough is killing me for more than 4 years. Why is God punishing me? Are you sure that I will come round soon." Again the rubrics are "fear extravagance of" and "business talks of". Will you again prescribe Opium 30 to cure his chronic cough? What idiocy is it that his cough can be cured on mental symptoms alone? Are not prominent homoeopaths like Segal misguiding their fellow students? Interpretation of the mentality and personality of a patient changes from man to man. Write down the sentences (what I said about this patient a moment ago) in a piece of paper and ask your fellow homoeopaths to interpret the underlying rubrics and their medicines. I am quite sure that the homoeopaths will not be able to reach (according to the 'mental symptom only' criteria) a unanimous conclusion about the patient mental rubric. The possible rubrics about the patient are: fearing extravagance, frugal, business minded, dejected, financially troubled, loving and caring, fear of future misfortune, dutiful, excessive sense duty, intolerance, wanting recognition (he speaks of his presentation in a manner to uphold his position), etc. Is there any fixed standard of plucking rubrics unanimously (I mean all the homoeopaths will be able to select the rubrics and medicines unanimously)? In this regard, I will opine that choosing medicines on mental symptoms alone is itself faulty. These medicines selected (ignoring the physical symptoms, hereditary history, past history, causation, prolonged exposure to noxious influence, etc) on mental symptoms alone are against Hahnemann's protocol of the 'Totality of Symptoms'.

What types of fallacy are these authors suffering from? What thing has inspired such diversion from the real teaching of Hahnemann? Indeed, it is some overenthusiastic authors' failure to grab the compatibility of Hahnemann's philosophy with the modern biological discoveries. Even in the 21st century, the immunological features of homoeopathic medicines are still unexplored. We know very little about how our medicines affect the nervous system, cardiovascular system, immune system, endocrine system, respiratory, reproductive system, etc. Regretfully, we still have not been able to establish relationship between homoeopathy and other branches of medical science such as anesthesiology, cardiology, dentistry, dermatology, epidemiology, endocrinology, gastroenterology, geriatrics, gynecology, hematology, hepatology, neurology, nephrology, obstretics, oncology, ophthalmology, optometry, orthopedics, pathology, Otorhinolaryngology, pediatrics, prophylaxis, psychiatry, pulmonology, radiology, Rheumatology, urology, etc. In a letter to Hering, Hahnemann wrote, "The time of the students should not be wasted with anatomical subtleties, not should botany or chemistry be carried too far."[108] But we need not be misguided by this statement. Hahnemann was upset with the animosity of the medical frontiers of his era. Moreover, he thought that his concepts like *vital force*, vital principles, vital functions, etc can, in no way, be proved in the laboratory. Also the homoeo-physicians who do not have without much knowledge of anatomy and biology could bring innumerous stunning results of cure by simply matching the disease-symptoms with the medicine-symptoms. So, it was quite normal that Hahnemann would make this statement.

Today, homoeopathy is a winning and competing science. We need to depend on science more and more because our science is the most complex one and we must make our science more acceptable with more scientific proofs. If we want to prove why and how homoeopathy can cure without putting your immune under extra pressure and why allopathy cannot, science can help us in this regard more than anything else. Now, where should we start integrating scientific findings into the science of Homoeopathy? Obviously, it is the materia medica which is full of lifeless accounts of symptoms. Almost all the homoeopaths tirelessly endeavor to match the drug symptoms with the disease symptoms without having any deeper knowledge of how and to what extent the selected medicines cure the disease. In this book, I will discuss few medicines and how their immunological properties can help curing diseases in order to exemplify what our materia medica should look like.

---

[108] Hahnemann, "Letter to Hering"
http://homeoint.org/books4/bradford/chapter68.htm

10
EXPLORATION OF THERAPEUTICS OF ARNICA MONT IN TERMS OF HAHNEMANN'S POSTULATION

Arnica Montana is an intensely toxic ethnobotanical flowering plant, found in Europe, which belongs to the sunflower family. Arnica extract contains essential oils, fatty acids, thymol, pseudoguaianolide sesquiterpene lactones and flavanone glycosides. The main toxic ingredient of Arnica extract is helenalin ($C15H18O4$), an anti-inflammatory (?) sesquiterpene lactone. The molar mass of Helenalin is 262.305 g•mol−1¬. Traditionally, Arnica Montana has been used by ethnic people as an anti-inflammatory herbal medicine for centuries. In an article, Marysia Kratimenos claims that "generations of Swiss mountain guides chewed arnica leaves to prevent fatigue induced by climbing…the dried leaves were used as a substitute for tobacco, hence its common name of mountain tobacco".[109] The use of Arnica compounds in popular cosmetics and anti-inflammatory ointment has been the cause of many researches and investigations on its toxicity and potential health risks. The US Food and Drug Administration has declared Arnica Montana as an unsafe herb because of two unidentified toxic compounds, found in arnica extracts, which are responsible for inducing "severe gastroenteritis, nervous disturbance, changes in pulse rate, intense muscular weakness, collapse, and death".[110]

---

[109] Marysia Kratimenos. "Arnica montana", British Homoeopathic Association. https://www.britishhomeopathic.org/charity/how-we-can-help/articles/homeopathic-medicines/a/arnica-montana/
[110] Monice Zondlo Fiume, "Final Report on the Safety Assessment of Arnica Montana Extract and Arnica Montana", International Journal of Toxicology, 20(Suppl. 2):1–11, 2001

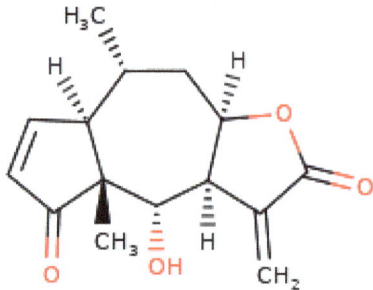

Helenalin ($C_{15}H_{18}O_4$)

Lethal Index: The median lethal dose or LD50 for Arnica Montana varies according to the routes of administration. For rabbits, the dermal LD50 of arnica resinoid was >5 g/kg, whereas the oral LD50 was >20 ml/kg.[111] It is soluble in water and insoluble in mineral oil. The LD50 for a single ip dose of helenalin and other toxic sesquiterpene lactones, the active toxic ingredient of Arnica extracts, for mice was 43 mg/kg".[112] Some studies found Helenalin as mutagenic.

Drug Pathology: Arnica extracts taken internally can cause severe gastroenteritis and internal bleeding of the digestive tract, shortness of breath (dyspnea), nervous disturbance, palpitation of heart, changes in pulse rate, muscular weakness and even death. Furthermore, the increased level of liver enzymes after oral administration of Arnica extract indicates that it is hepatotoxic also. Researchers unanimously agreed on the cyto-toxicity of helenalin. In an article, "Acute toxicity of helenalin in BDF1 mice", Chapman et al reported that "a single ip injection of 25 mg helenalin/kg increased serum alanine aminotransferase (ALT), lactate dehydrogenase (LDH), urea nitrogen (BUN), and sorbitol dehydrogenase within 6 hr of treatment".[113] Though

---

[111] Monice Zondlo Fiume, "Final Report on the Safety Assessment of Arnica Montana Extract and Arnica Montana", International Journal of Toxicology, 20(Suppl. 2):1–11, 2001

[112] Chapman DE, Roberts GB, Reynolds DJ, Grippo AA, Holbrook DJ, Hall IH, Chaney SG, Chang J, Lee KH. "Acute toxicity of helenalin in BDF1 mice." PUBMED NCBI. Fundam Appl Toxicol. 1988 Feb;10(2):302-12
https://www.ncbi.nlm.nih.gov/pubmed/3356317

[113] Chapman et al. "Acute toxicity of helenalin in BDF1 mice".
https://www.ncbi.nlm.nih.gov/pubmed/3356317

there is not any well-explained 'mechanism of helenalin-toxicity', Chapman's report can help us to grab the basic process of the toxic influence of helenalin on cells and other biological functions. The increased LDH in blood is a clear indicator of the possible tissue damage of the host cell. It is not known how helenalin molecules cause damages to the tissue. But the increase in the level of LDH in blood shows that helenalin-molecule's contact with host cell causes damages in some unknown ways. So, if the dose of helenalin is large enough to mix into the blood flow and reach the liver, it causes damages to both liver and kidneys. Consequently, it gives rise to the levels of serum alanine aminotransferase (ALT) and urea nitrogen (BUN). The immune-response to tissue-damage caused by helenalin is similar to that of accidental tissue-damage. The immune-responses in both cases are the same inflammatory response which is induced by any tissue damage in injury. The similarity between helenalin-caused tissue damage and injury-related tissue damage is further proved by the fact that "multiple helenalin exposures, ip injection of 25 mg helenalin/kg for 3 days, increased differential polymorphonuclear leukocyte counts and decreased lymphocyte counts".[114] In their article, Chapman et al further report that "three concurrent days of diethyl maleate (DEM) pretreatment (3.7 mmol DEM/kg, 0.5 hr before helenalin treatment) significantly increased the toxicity of helenalin exposure".[115] In another article, "Final Report on the Safety Assessment of Arnica Montana Extract and Arnica Montana", Monice Zondlo Fiume claimed that dermal application of arnica tincture form (70% from 1 part flower and 10 parts ethanol), can result in edematous and vesicular eczema. Arnica dermatitis is an allergic contact dermatitis, i.e., a delayed-reaction type IV allergy. The allergic dermatitis is caused by the helenanolides, sesquiterpene lactones found in the flowers of A. Montana. However, the basic steps in the mechanism of helenalin toxicity are as following:

---

[114] Chapman et al. "Acute toxicity of helenalin in BDF1 mice". https://www.ncbi.nlm.nih.gov/pubmed/3356317
[115] Chapman et al. "Acute toxicity of helenalin in BDF1 mice". https://www.ncbi.nlm.nih.gov/pubmed/3356317

THE SCIENCE OF HOMOEOPATHIC IMMUNOLOGY

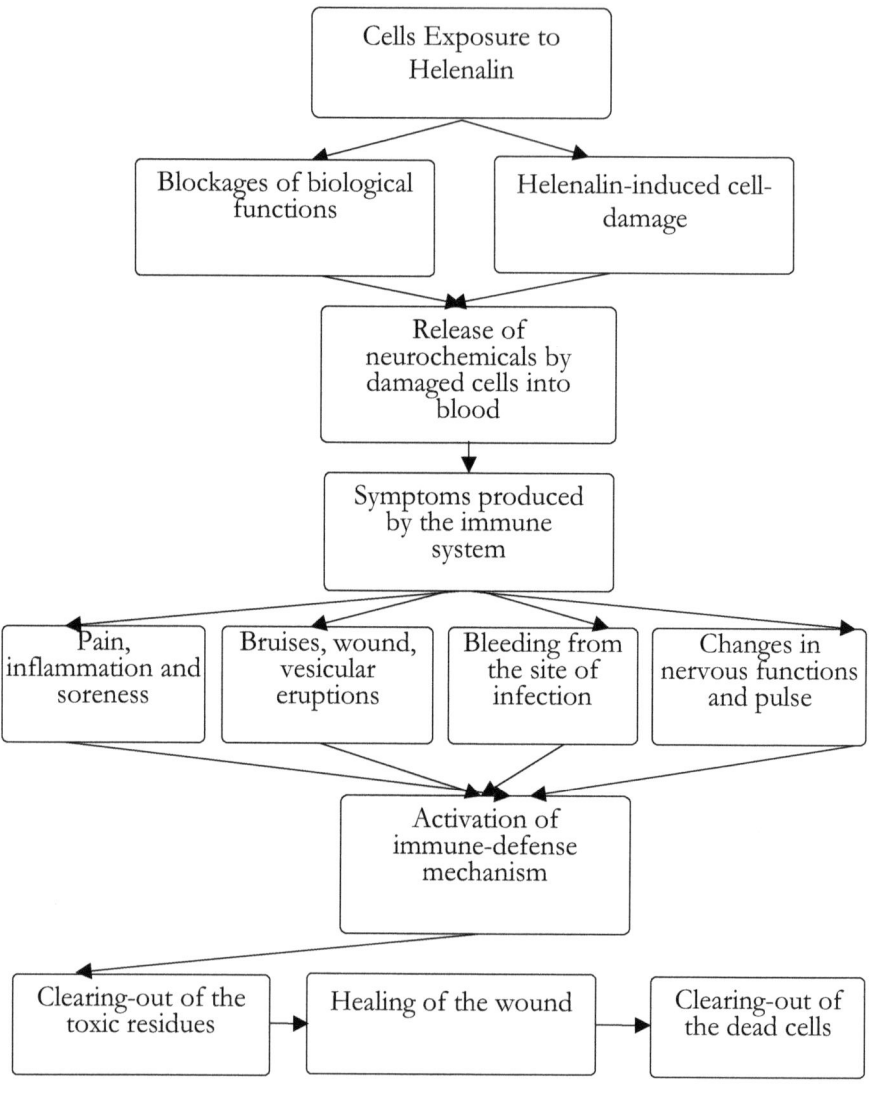

Pharmacokinetics: No specific research has yet been led on the absorption, distribution, metabolism, and excretion of Arnica Montana Extract and Arnica Montana. But it is supposed that molecules of Helenalin and other sesquiterpene lactones are primarily neutralized by its binding to the cells and subsequent cell-damage. Since the cell-damage, caused by Helenalin molecules, is similar to the tissue injury, caused by thrashing, Helenalin-induced cell-damage invites the phagocytes to the affected part. So, the large portion of the administered arnica extracts are consumed and cleared out by the phagocytosis of the host organism. If the dose is large enough to mix into the blood, a part of it is stored and decomposed in the liver. Also, the kidney and the perspiration mechanism of the body play some selective roles to clear out the neutralized and decomposed helenalin molecules with urine and stool.

Therapeutic Features: Though Arnica Montana is well-known for its anti-inflammatory properties, researchers have not been able so far to explain its mechanism of action. It means that scientists do not know how Arnica extract cures inflammation. In this regard, Hahnemann's postulation of 'Threat *Momentum*' can help us to understand the anti-inflammatory of Arnica Montana. Indeed, the drug pathology and the therapeutic individuality of Arnica extracts are quite contradictory to each other. Arnica Montana was reported to be used as anti-inflammatory ingredients in more than 100 cosmetic formulations across a wide range of product types. On the other hands, almost all the researches which were led on the safety of using Arnica extracts in cosmetics claimed that it is cytotoxic, inflammatory and mutagenic. Referring to these two contradictory properties of Arnica Montana, G Lyss et al says that "while [sesquiterpene lactones] affect various cellular processes, current data do not fully explain how sesquiterpene lactones exert their anti-inflammatory effect".[116] In another article the same authors says, "The sesquiterpene lactone helenalin is a potent anti-inflammatory drug whose molecular mechanism of action remains unclear despite numerous investigations."[117] There is another contradiction in the anti-platelet activities of Arnica extracts. Most of the safety reports on the Arnica extracts claim that sesquiterpene lactones, which are found in Arnica extracts, cause severe damages to host cells and such cell-damages ultimately result into severe gastroenteritis and internal bleeding of the digestive tract. But in an article, "Comparison of cytotoxic and anti-platelet activities of polyphenolic extracts from Arnica montana flowers and Juglans regia husks", J Rywaniak et al reports that "[polyphenolic compounds, found in Arnica extracts] exert[s] protective effects on haemostasis and have a particular influence on blood platelets".[118] Let's see how Hahnemann's postulation can take us of this

---

[116] Lyss G, Schmidt TJ, Merfort I, Pahl HL. "Helenalin, an anti-inflammatory sesquiterpene lactone from Arnica, selectively inhibits transcription factor NF-kappaB." PUBMED. NCBI. https://www.ncbi.nlm.nih.gov/pubmed/9348104
[117] Lyss G, Schmidt TJ, Merfort I, Pahl HL "The anti-inflammatory sesquiterpene lactone helenalin inhibits the transcription factor NF-kappaB by directly targeting" https://www.ncbi.nlm.nih.gov/pubmed/9837931
[118] Rywaniak J1, Luzak B, Podsedek A, Dudzinska D, Rozalski M, Watala C. "Comparison of cytotoxic and anti-platelet activities of polyphenolic extracts from Arnica montana flowers and Juglans regia husks", PUBMED, NCBI. https://www.ncbi.nlm.nih.gov/pubmed/24679412

confusion. We should read the postulation again:

> If the immune system (*vital force*) detects two (almost) similar threats simultaneously, the immune responses (actions of vital principles) which are metered by the severer one consider both threats as one qualitatively unitary target and treat them with the same defense and recuperative strategies. During the immune responses in action, the less severe infection will be cured faster than the severer one. (I have already mentioned it earlier in this article)

In fact, this postulation was essentially Hahnemann's attempt to manipulate a biological phenomenon therapeutically. For thousands of years, human civilization knew that if a living organism is challenged by any hostile agent, it will grow (short term and long term) biological defense against the hostile presence. With Jenner's invention of pox-vaccine, men, for the first time in human history, started to handle such biological phenomenon as preventive (prophylaxis) of diseases. But Hahnemann proposed that this self-defense of living-organism can be handled to cure diseases also. Indeed, such claim about the therapeutic use of organism's self-defense was confusing for his contemporary medical scholars because they did not know much about Warner's *Momentum* which Hahnemann introduced in the Jupitar analogy in Aphorism 26 of the Organon:

> Why does brilliant Jupiter disappear in the light of dawn to the optic nerve of the beholder? Because a very similar though greater power, the light of dawning day, acts upon the optic nerve.[119]

> In the living organism a weaker dynamic affection is permanently extinguished by a stronger one, which, through different in nature, nevertheless greatly resembles it in expression.[120]

Even today, medical scholars have failed to understand the proper meaning of this Jupitar Analogy. They are mostly confused by the maze how it is possible to cure the pain and inflammation of a finger (which have been thrashed by a heavy and large hammer) with substances (like Helenalin in Arnica Mont) which will rather cause the same pain and inflammation. Indeed, such maze is the layman's less intelligent perception of a more complex therapeutic phenomenon. Whenever Hahnemann attempted to explain the mechanism of action of his newly invented medicine, he advocated about challenging the *vital force* (or immune system) with a stronger but easily subsiding threatening agent. Please note here the two points: a.

---

[119] Hahnemann, the Organon of Medicine. Aphorism 26
[120] Hahnemann, the Organon of Medicine. Aphorism 26

stronger threat and b. easily subsiding threat. Though Hahnemann's postulation was quite reasonable, the therapeutic effect of stronger but easily subsiding threatening agent was confusing for the medical scholars because they are confronted with the question: "Though diluting the toxic substance makes it easily disposable (easily subsiding) for the immune system, how does it become strong enough to evoke the desired immune response?" We have explained earlier that the sole target of a homoeopathic medicine is to create the *threat momentum* which will be able to evoke the immune system to initiate the doctor-desired immune response. We have shown that the *threat momentum* (or Warner's *Momentum*) for any specific amount of toxic substance is higher in any area which is nearer to the Central Nervous System. It means that the smallest amount of Helenalin which can easily terrorize the immune system and evoke the counter immune responses if administered on the tongue can stir nothing if administered on any inflammatory part of the leg. For the same reason, while the allopaths apply Arnica-balms (which contain 40 percent arnica-extract of the main ingredients) on any bruises, wounds, inflammatory-parts of the organs, etc, the homoeopaths manipulate the smallest diluted amount of Helenalin to reduce the inflammation. Moreover, the homoeopathic tactic of administering the lowest amount of helenalin-molecules renders several benefits for the therapeutic effects:

a. The homoeopathic tactic of administering the lowest amount of helenalin-molecules does not exert any lethal effects on the immune systems.

b. The homoeopathic method of administering the least amount of helenalin-molecules does not suppress/oppose what the immune system wants to perform against inflammation or inflammatory agent.

c. Rather, the homoeopathic use of Arnica Mont create a threatening environment which provokes the immune system to take effective measures against the inflammation, inflammatory agents, cell-damages, etc freely.

d. Since administering the least amount of Arnica molecules at the most ideal route creates the most effective threat *momentum*, the immune response generated by the immune system (against those molecules) abstractly can address any inflammation or threat in the body.

e. So, whereas the allopathic external application of Arnica ointment can cure only external inflammation, the homoeopathic application of the least of amount of medication at the most effective route can cure the inflammation or damages of internal organs.

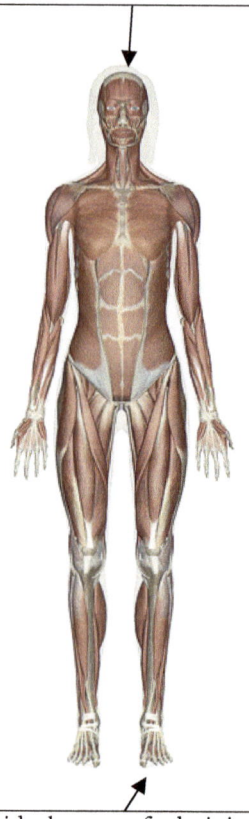

The most ideal route of administration where the least amount of medicinal molecules can create the desired threat momentum

The least ideal route of administration where the largest amount of medicinal molecules can create the desired threat momentum

The abovementioned explanation of the anti-inflammatory effect of Arnica Montana was, for the first time in human history, narrated by Hahnemann. His contemporary society as well as the modern scholars' failure to understand the scientific essences (and biological evidences) of Hahnemann's philosophy has, so far, made them keep wondering how the hell "sesquiterpene lactones (the active inflammatory ingredient of Arnica extracts) exert their anti-inflammatory effects."[121] Hahnemann's treatment

---

[121] Lyss G, Schmidt TJ, Merfort I, Pahl HL. "Helenalin, an anti-inflammatory

strategy of manipulating the immune system's hostility against toxic substances for curing human sufferings has given Arnica an important medicine which can be used to get rid of a good number of sufferings. Now, the mystery of the anti-inflammatory effect of Arnica Montana (though Helenalin) has been dissolved through Hahnemann's Postulation and Warner's *Momentum*.

---

sesquiterpene lactone from Arnica, selectively inhibits transcription factor NF-kappaB." PUBMED. NCBI. https://www.ncbi.nlm.nih.gov/pubmed/9348104

11
SUCCUSSION AND HIGH POTENCY: CENTURY-OLD INJUSTICE DONE TO HAHNEMANN

What is 'succussion' really? I think, it is one of those homoeopathic concepts which have suffered century-old injustice, inflicted from both the homoeopathic and allopathic medical sectors. The allopathic school will not acknowledge the scientific essence of 'succussion' because of either their failure to perceive it or their intentional animosity against homeopathy. But how is it possible that the homoeopaths too so far misunderstood Hahnemann? Can you see anything abnormal in the following definitions of 'succussion?' Dr. Manish Bhatia, an Indian Homoeopath, defined 'succussion' as one of three steps (i.e. Serial dilution, Succussion and Trituration) of the preparation of homoeopathic medicines. Please note that for Dr. Manish 'serial dilution' is meant to reduce toxicity and 'succussion' and 'trituration' are the "methods by which mechanical energy is delivered to our preparations in order to imprint the pharmacological message of the original drug upon the molecules of the diluents".[122] Indeed, Dr. Manish is one of those careless readers who intentionally want to read the Organon of Medicine as a medieval, but still necessary, medical script and therefore miss the scientific essences. Why will a homeopath with a little bit of common sense miss the very necessary relationship between 'dilution' and 'succussion'? It is very easy to perceive that 'succussion' or 'violent shaking' is a crucial step (in preparing a perfect dilution) which is performed to diffuse the medicinal molecules equally all over the dilutant. Homoeopaths like Dr. Manish will never understand the simple science behind 'succussion' or 'potentization' because they have failed to delve deep into the linguistic deficiency which Hahnemann suffered so violently in his era. I wonder if Dr. Manish ever read the Organon of Medicine carefully. I do not know which lines from the Organon pushed

---

[122] Dr. Manish Bhatia, "Preparation of Drugs & Homeopathic Scales of Dilution", https://hpathy.com/pharmacology/preparation-of-drugs-homeopathic-scales-of-dilution/

him to make such comments. Who told him that 'succussion' and 'trituration' are meant "to deliver mechanical energy to homoeopathic preparations" and "to imprint the pharmacological message of the original drug upon the molecules of the diluents"? What mechanical energy (?) and pharmacological message (?) is he talking of? Did Hahnemann also say so? Let's endeavor to understand how Hahnemann himself perceived 'succussion' and 'trituration'.

For Hahnemann, the first and foremost criterion for any substance to be considered as the raw-material of homoeopathic medicines is that it must be harmful and poisonous enough to make changes in the vital functions (biological functions) and therefore, to initiate immune response. Initially, he used to prescribe the poisonous substances in raw forms. But later he started giving diluted medicines in order to minimize the poisonous effects of the medicines. Obviously, Hahnemann, a man of common sense, was wise enough to shake the medicine-dilution well and violently before preparing the potencies so that he could get the desired quantity of the equally diffused medicinal molecules. Astonishingly he noticed that the diluted medicines or the smaller doses of the medicines work even better than what the larger doses do. So he tried to give an explanation of this natural phenomenon of the increased-efficacy-smaller-doses in his own way. He declared that the diluted medicinal molecules become more powerful or energized with some pharmacological energies because of the succussion or violent shaking. In Aphorism 128, Hahnemann mentions 'succussion' as following:

The latest discoveries, as well as earlier ones, have shown that crude medicinal substances when taken by the prover to test their characteristic effects do not express the full range of their latent hidden powers nearly as much as those taken in high dilutions correctly potentized by trituration and succussion. By this simple process the virtues hidden and, as it were, lying dormant in their crude state are developed to an unbelievable degree and roused to activity.

Modern laboratories have still failed to discover those energies which Hahnemann mentioned in his explanation. So, was Hahnemann wrong? Indeed, Hahnemann was a careful empiricist. He observed anything carefully before theorizing it. When he attempted to use diluted medicines in order for minimizing the poisonous effects, he astonishingly noticed that the efficacy of his medicines rather increased. Indeed, Hahnemann did not have any logical explanation of this apparently contradicting phenomenon. For him, the only possible reason behind these apparently contradicting features of the diluted medicine was the violent shaking (which he called 'succussion') which was performed during the preparation of the dilution. Hahnemann defines the mystery of the efficacy of diluted substances in the footnote of Aphorism 269:

Similarly, by the trituration of a medicinal substance and the succussion of its solution (dynamization, potentization) the medicinal forces lying hidden in it are developed and uncovered more and more, and the material is itself spiritualized, if one may use that expression.[123]

Was this explanation of Hahnemann scientific? Nope! While providing the explanation of the increased efficacy of smaller doses, Hahnemann made two mistakes (certainly I will stay respectful to this great scientist of the medical history): a. first, the 'succussion' (or violent shaking) theory as the enhancer or liberator of medicinal forces never could have satisfied the rational minds, b. second, he claimed the medicines could be potentized infinitely. The single reason which is responsible for both of these two mistakes of Hahnemann was his assumption that toxic properties of crude substance are spiritual (or non-physical) and they can be transferred to other substances (as magnetism can be transferred to iron). For him dilution though succussion and trituration reduces the substance's toxic properties and increases the spiritual medicinal properties. So, he did not put much attention to his contemporary Amedeo Avogadro's claim about the constancy of the number of molecules in molecular weight of a substance. Indeed, Hahnemann failed to acknowledge the toxic properties of a substance at the molecular level. Also, he had no credible explanation of how the reduced dose of the toxic substance works more effectively except the vague (?) 'succussion' theory of liberating 'spirit-like medicinal force' with violent rhythmical shaking.

Earlier in this paper, we have leant how knowledge about modern immunological science can explain the effectiveness of smaller doses to induce therapeutic immune responses against any pathogenic condition. Though Hahnemann's philosophy of the 'man' was a surprising abstractive essence of the immune system, he was not familiar with its specific features. May be, if he knew about the specific immune responses against specific medicinal molecules, if he knew that the tongue is the most innervated organ of the body, that the oral route of administration is the highest immunity area of human body, that substances' toxic properties cannot be transferred to the molecules of dilutants, that crude substances' toxicity does not turn into any spiritual medicinal energy, that immune system's defense against the molecules of the crude toxic substance does all the magic cures and that several hundred molecules of the toxic crude substance can infuriate the whole immune system if they are administered at highly immune areas i.e. tongue, mouth, etc, I am quite sure that a wise scholar like Hahnemann could explain the pharmacodynamics of his diluted medicines more eloquently than I did in this paper. So, succussion is nothing but an attempt to disentangle the molecules of any substance by breaking through the intermolecular energy by manipulating the collisions between the particles of solutions and those of medicinal substances, so that the lowest but the effective doses can be determined. If there is any better technology for breaking the medicinal substances into molecules, it can replace the process of Succussion.

---

[123] Hahnemann, the Organon of Medicine. Aphorism 26

What do you think what Hahnemann would do if he knew that the possibility of the presence of medicinal molecules in the higher potencies is almost zero? Unlike some of the overenthusiastic homoeopaths, Hahnemann was never driven by the irrational romantic utopian love for the high potencies, as in his article, "Hahnemann and High Potency", Peter Morrell says, "Hahnemann rejected the use of higher potencies [not only] because he was opposed to the sort of quasi-mystical ideas some of Kent's predecessors were keen on".[124] As discussed earlier in this paper, a substance must be toxic in order to be homeopathically medicinal. As per the laws of physics, if a substance is considered toxic, its molecules also retain the toxic features of that substance. So, it is quite explainable why the lower potencies (up to 30th potency) work so quickly and effectively. The toxic molecules in the dilutant do all those miracles of homoeopathic medicines. But if it is proved in the laboratory that higher potencies contain almost none of the toxic molecules, how will they provoke the desired immune responses? Was not Hahnemann aware of the possible absence of medicinal molecules in higher potencies? It is very much difficult to speak for sure whether Hahnemann was aware of it or not. But evidences show that he was anxious about setting the limit of higher potencies. In his article, Peter Morrell assessed Hahnemann's use of potency as following:

> Hahnemann himself felt, in 1829, the urgent necessity of a limit in potentisation and declared the ultimate degree of dilution to be the 30th centesimal potency.[125]

However, records show that he had once suggested prescribing potencies which are higher than the 30th in 1825. He suggested prescribing the 60th potency of Thuja for gonorrhea. Nonetheless, his doubt in higher potencies is shown in one of his letters to to Dr Schréter, of Lemberg, of the 12 Sept 1829:

> I do not approve of your potentising medicines higher than to XII and XXII [my emphasis] - there must be a limit to the matter, it cannot go on indefinitely. But by definitely deciding that homoeopathic medicines should be diluted and potentised up to X (= 30 CH) a homogeneous process arises in the cures of all homoeopaths and if they describe a cure, we are able to work after them in the same degree, since they are operating with the same tools as we are. Then our enemies cannot reproach us with all having nothing definite, no fixed standard.[126]

---

[124] Peter Morrell, "Hahnemann and High Potency", http://www.homeoint.org/morrell/articles/pm_highp.htm
[125] Peter Morrell, "Hahnemann and High Potency
[126] Bradford (1895) Life and Letters of Hahnemann, Jain

Please note the underlined part of the abovementioned quotation. Possibly, he was not familiar with the knowledge of molecular physics available in his contemporary era. But the assertion that "there must be a limit to the matter, it cannot go on indefinitely" shows that Hahnemann was anxious about the actual presence of the medicinal substance in the highly potentized medicines. In his article, "Hahnemann and High Potency", Peter Morrell have analyzed the potencies prescribed by Hahnemann during the last years of his life and shown that the potencies prescribed by Hahnemann are mostly below the 30th potency, as he says,

> Finally, we can safely say that Hahnemann at the end of his career mainly used potencies 12, 18, 24 and 30 and that this comprised some 81% of his total prescribing. If we then add potencies 6 and 9, we cover some 94% of his total prescribing.[127]

Peter Morrell further claims:

"The final phase of his prescribing runs from 1830 to 1843, comprising 27.7% 30c, 25.6% 18c and 25.2% 6c. Also during this phase (from c1840 onwards) he makes increasing use of olfaction and the LM potencies."

"Those homoeopaths who can with honesty say they use mainly potencies 12, 18, 24 and 30 can truly call themselves Hahnemannian. The rest cannot."

Let's see the number of molecules which the single drops of the potencies contains. In this regard, we will use to equation to calculate the molecules. Compare the following two tables. You will see that almost 60% of the potencies prescribed by Hahnemann contained significant number of medicinal molecules.

$$N_{mt} = \frac{6.022 \times 10^{23}}{mol \times 15.4324} \times \frac{1}{10^6} \times \frac{1}{500^n} \times \frac{1}{100^n}$$

Where,
N_{mt} = Number of molecules in 1 drop of LM mother tincture
(The dilution made from 1 gram of crude substance)
500 drops = 25 ml
1 gram = 15.4324 grain

---

[127] Peter Morrell, "Hahnemann and High Potency

| LM POTENCY | NUMBER of Molecules in Medicines in 1 drop of LM potency |||||
	Sulphur (S) 32g/mol	Merc S (Hg.2NO3.2H3N) 358g/mol	Natrum Mur (NaCl) 58g/mol	Arnica-Helenalin ($C_{15}H_{18}O_4$) 262.305 g/mol	Silicea (SiO_2) 60.08 g/mol
1	3.76×10^{11}	3.36×10^{10}	2.07×10^{11}	4.59×10^{10}	2.0×10^{11}
2	7.5×10^6	6.67×10^5	4.1×10^6	9.19×10^5	4.01×10^6
3	150	13.4	83.06	18.38	80.29
4	.0030	.00026	.00166	.00036	.0016
5	0	0	0	0	0
6	0	0	0	0	0
7	0	0	0	0	0
8	0	0	0	0	0
9	0	0	0	0	0
10	0	0	0	0	0

The number of molecules in 100ml of nth centesimal potency will be counted with the following equation:

$$Num = \frac{6.022 \times 10^{23}}{mol \times 100^n}$$

Where,
Num= Number of molecules in 1ml of nth potency

Centesimal POTENCY	NUMBER of Molecules in Medicines in 1 ml of Centesimal potency				
	Sulphur (S) 32g/mol	Merc S (Hg.2NO3. 2H3N) 358g/mol	Natrum Mur (NaCl) 58g/mol	Arnica-Helenalin ($C_{15}H_{18}O_4$) 262.305 g/mol	Silicea (SiO_2) 60.08 g/mol
1C	1.88×10^{20}	1.68×10^{19}	1.03×10^{20}	2.29×10^{19}	1.01×10^{20}
2C	1.88×10^{18}	1.68×10^{17}	1.03×10^{18}	2.29×10^{17}	1.01×10^{18}
3C	1.88×10^{16}	1.68×10^{15}	1.03×10^{16}	2.29×10^{15}	1.01×10^{16}
4C	1.88×10^{14}	1.68×10^{13}	1.03×10^{14}	2.29×10^{13}	1.01×10^{14}
5C	1.88×10^{12}	1.68×10^{11}	1.03×10^{12}	2.29×10^{11}	1.01×10^{12}
6C	1.88×10^{10}	1.68×10^{9}	1.03×10^{10}	2.29×10^{9}	1.01×10^{10}
7C	1.88×10^{8}	1.68×10^{7}	1.03×10^{8}	2.29×10^{7}	1.01×10^{8}
8C	1.88×10^{6}	1.68×10^{5}	1.03×10^{6}	2.29×10^{5}	1.01×10^{6}
9C	1.88×10^{4}	1.68×10^{3}	1.03×10^{4}	2.29×10^{3}	1.01×10^{4}
10C	1.88×10^{2}	1.68×10^{1}	1.03×10^{2}	2.29×10^{1}	1.01×10^{2}
11C	1.88	.168	1.03	.229	1.01
12C	.018	.0068	.0103	.0029	.01
18C	0	0	0	0	0
24C	0	0	0	0	0
30C	0	0	0	0	0

Now, you can be sure of how toxic molecules of homoeopathic medicines work. Just to remind you again that there are thousands of chemorecetors in the oral cavity. Simply the tongue itself is equipped with 5 thousands to 20 thousands taste buds each of which contains 50-150 receptors cells. So, the tongue is innervated with 250000 to 3 million of chemoreceptors. If we take the receptors on the walls of oral cavities into consideration, the number of chemoreceptors in the oral cavity may reach several billions. These chemoreceptors detect:

Toxic or hazardous chemicals in the internal or external environment of the human body (e.x. chemotherapy) and transmits that information to the central nervous system, (and rarely the peripheral nervous system), in order to expel the biologically active toxins from the blood, and prevent further consumption of alcohol and/or other acutely toxic recreational intoxicants.[128]

However, you must reread the earlier parts of this paper in order to learn what happens when these millions of chemoreceptors detect the toxic molecules on the tongue. Finally, I cannot but make a humble challenge to my readers. Once, one of the homeopaths I personally know said that the longer the patient's suffering under allopathic treatment, the more intensive the ecstasy of curing is. The ecstasy of curing a patient, who has already run away from the allopathic medical system and taken refuge to a homoeopath, compares to nothing because the tasteless and colorless negligible pills of homoeopathic medicines have seldom failed to win a prestigious chair for you above the MBBSs, FRCSs, etc. Hahnemann expressed this joy of winning over the traditional medical sector as following: "Changes that come to material substances, specially the medicinal…are so incredible that may be compared to miracles, and is a reason of joy that those changes belong to Homoeopathy".[129] It is really miraculous that the poisonous substances after "trituration of non-medicinal powder, agitation of non-medicinal fluid" become so powerful that they can easily outweigh their allopathic counterparts. But is it really that miracle beyond any scientific explanation? Is Homoeopathy really a pseudoscience which is incompatible with scientific methods? What about all those patients whom you cured with tiresome selections of medicines? What about all those thankful eyes of your patients? Are all those cures illusions in the name of treatment? The critics of Homoeopathy are, indeed, saying so. See what the British House of Commons Science and Technology Committee stated in an article in 2010: "In our view, the systematic reviews and meta-analyses conclusively demonstrate that homeopathic products perform no better than placebos. The Government shares our interpretation of the evidence".[130] There are many more of such claims which will outright go against your hard-earned achievements and your experiences of successes as a homoeopath. When you cured a patient whom the Allopathic medical system had already failed, he/she would bring more patients simply being driven by gratefulness, but those critics will negate the whole event of the treatment and cure of the patient with the following points:

1. The intensive consultation process of homoeopathic case-taking (that is, the placebo effect) might have cured the disease.

---

[128] Wikipidea "Chemoreceptor", https://en.wikipedia.org/wiki/Chemoreceptor
[129] This speech of Hahnemann is collected from internet source
[130] Collected from the internet.

2. The care, compassion, concern, and reassurance of a homoeopath have partial curative effects on the patients

3. The Homoeopathic medicines did nothing to the patients; rather they came round because the body's ability to get well on its own.

4. Allopathic medicines which are taken along with the homeopathic medicines might cure the patients.

5. Cessation of the allopathic medicines might relieve the patients of the adverse effects of those medicines and the credit may go to the homoeopathic medicines.

Look, the abovementioned points are their so-called scientific explanations of how homoeopathy might work. Criminals always leave some evidences behind. Their explanations of how homeopathy works, surprisingly, unveil their dark intentions of hiding the truth and perpetuating the sufferings of thousands of the unfortunates. When some mercenary-writers negate the homoeopathic medical industry and its realities of cure, there must be something dark and fishy working behind those bulldogs which are being pampered for their barking to distract the public focus away from the reality. So here is a challenge for those critics to prove the efficacy of homoeopathy. Find 100 patients, with allergic itching and urticaria, who are sensitive to various allergens. These patients must have to be treated with allopathic medicines for more than 5 years and subsequently have been failed to be cured permanently. Hence, those clowns must ensure that the followings of the five claims (of how homoeopathy works) must not happen to those patients:

a. Those clowns must testify that the allergic diseases of those patients will not be cured by any 'intensive consultation' process. If they claim that allergy can be cured by intensive consultation, they must cure 1 or 2 patients with skin allergy in support of their claim.

b. If they claim that skin allergy can be cured by 'care, compassion and reassurance', they must cure several patients in support of their claim. So, they must ensure that there must not be any patient (among those 100 participating patients) who can be cured by 'care, compassion and reassurance'. Otherwise, if the credit of cure goes to Homoeopathy, you must not lament.

c. If the body with the support of the allopathic medicines has been failing to heal on its own for more than 5 years, is it possible that the body will cure it miraculously during the homoeopathic medication period?

d. They must ensure that the patients will not take any subsidiary allopathic medicines. Moreover, the medicines which have been failing for more than 5 years will not stand up on their feet and start working vigorously, as those clowns expect, to prove homoeopathy false.

e. If you stop allopathic medications for those patients on your own, the homoeopaths will consider it as a favor.

Now, take those patients to one or several experienced homoeopaths and analyze the rate of cures by homoeopathy in comparison with allopathic medicines. The obvious is that what the allopaths fear even to dream is possible in homoeopathy. Do you dare taking the challenge? Or will you still acknowledge Homoeopathy as an unveiled science?

BIBLIOGRAPHY

Adam Felman. "Everything you need to know about infections", Medical News Today. https://www.medicalnewstoday.com/articles/196271.php

Ann Jerome Croce. "The Thought Behind the Action - Understanding suppression", National Center for Homoeopathy. https://www.homeopathycenter.org/homeopathy-today/thought-behind-action-understanding-suppression

Ann Jerome Croce. "The Thought Behind the Action - Miasms: Psora, Syphilis, Sycosis". National Center for Homoeopathy. https://www.homeopathycenter.org/homeopathy-today/thought-behind-action-miasms-psora-syphilis-sycosis

BECHTEL, WILLIAM and ROBERT C. RICHARDSON. "Vitalism". In E. Craig (Ed.), Routledge Encyclopedia of Philosophy. London: Routledge. http://mechanism.ucsd.edu/teaching/philbio/vitalism.htm

Bradford (1895) Life and Letters of Hahnemann, Jain

Brommer B, Engel O, Kopp MA, Watzlawick R, Müller S, Prüss H, Chen Y, DeVivo MJ, Finkenstaedt FW, Dirnagl U, Liebscher T, Meisel A, Schwab JM. Spinal cord injury-induced immune deficiency syndrome enhances infection susceptibility dependent on lesion level. Brain. 2016 Jan 10. https://www.ncbi.nlm.nih.gov/pmc/articles/PMC5014125/

C. Fookes. "Nonsteroidal anti-inflammatory drugs", Drugs. https://www.drugs.com/drug-class/nonsteroidal-anti-inflammatory-agents.html

Chapman DE, Roberts GB, Reynolds DJ, Grippo AA, Holbrook DJ, Hall IH, Chaney SG, Chang J, Lee KH. "Acute toxicity of helenalin in BDF1 mice." PUBMED NCBI. Fundam Appl Toxicol. 1988 Feb;10(2):302-12 https://www.ncbi.nlm.nih.gov/pubmed/3356317

Chapman et al. "Acute toxicity of helenalin in BDF1 mice". https://www.ncbi.nlm.nih.gov/pubmed/3356317

Daniel Eskinazi, "Homeopathy Re-revisited: Is Homeopathy Compatible With Biomedical Observations?" JAMA International Medicine. https://jamanetwork.com/journals/jamainternalmedicine/fullarticle/485127

Dantzer R, Wollman EE. "Relationships between the brain and the immune system". J Soc Biol. 2003;197(2):81-8 in NCBI https://www.ncbi.nlm.nih.gov/pubmed/12910622

David Little. "Miasms in Classical Miasms in Classical Homeopathy", Homoeo Academe Journal. https://sites.google.com/a/homoeoacademe.com/journal1/miasms-in-classical-homoeopathy-part-i-david-little

E A Farrington. A Supplement to Gross' Comparative Materia Medica. Volume 1. https://www.forgottenbooks.com/en/books/ASupplementtoGrossComparativeMateriaMedica_10663056

Haehl, Richard, Samuel Hahnemann, His Life and Work, Vol II, p. 148.

Irvine Loudon, "A brief history of homeopathy", JSRM https://www.ncbi.nlm.nih.gov/pmc/articles/PMC1676328/

Ke Ren and Ronald Dubner. "Interactions between the immune and nervous systems in pain", NCBI. https://www.ncbi.nlm.nih.gov/pmc/articles/PMC3077564/

Laura Foist. "*Vital force* Theory". Study. https://study.com/academy/lesson/vital-force-theory-definition-principals.html

Lyss G, Schmidt TJ, Merfort I, Pahl HL. "Helenalin, an anti-inflammatory sesquiterpene lactone from Arnica, selectively inhibits transcription factor NF-kappaB." PUBMED. NCBI. https://www.ncbi.nlm.nih.gov/pubmed/9348104

Lyss G, Schmidt TJ, Merfort I, Pahl HL "The anti-inflammatory sesquiterpene lactone helenalin inhibits the transcription factor NF-kappaB by directly targeting" https://www.ncbi.nlm.nih.gov/pubmed/9837931

Manish Bhatia, "Preparation of Drugs & Homeopathic Scales of Dilution", https://hpathy.com/pharmacology/preparation-of-drugs-homeopathic-scales-of-dilution/

Marysia Kratimenos. "Arnica montana", British Homoeopathic Association. https://www.britishhomeopathic.org/charity/how-we-can-help/articles/homeopathic-medicines/a/arnica-montana/

Mayo Clinic. "Whooping Cough". https://www.mayoclinic.org/diseases-conditions/whooping-cough/symptoms-causes/syc-20378973

Medicineplus. "What is pain?", US National Library of Medicine. https://medlineplus.gov/nondrugpainmanagement.html

Medicineplus. "Viral Infections", US National Library of Medicine. https://medlineplus.gov/viralinfections.html

Mohit Mathur. "The concept of miasm—evolution and present day perspective", Homeopathy (2009) 98, 177–180

Monice Zondlo Fiume, "Final Report on the Safety Assessment of Arnica Montana Extract and Arnica Montana", International Journal of Toxicology, 20(Suppl. 2):1–11, 2001

Nachum Dafny. "Chapter 6: Pain Principles", Neuroscience Online. https://nba.uth.tmc.edu/neuroscience/m/s2/chapter06.html

Peter Morrell, "Hahnemann and High Potency", http://www.homeoint.org/morrell/articles/pm_highp.htm

Rajan Sankaran, http://www.theothersong.com/international/sensation-method-in-homoeopathy/

Rywaniak J, Luzak B, Podsedek A, Dudzinska D, Rozalski M, Watala C. "Comparison of cytotoxic and anti-platelet activities of polyphenolic extracts from Arnica montana flowers and Juglans regia husks", PUBMED, NCBI. https://www.ncbi.nlm.nih.gov/pubmed/24679412

Samuel Hahnemann. "Hahnemann Quotes", http://homeopatia.bvs.br/en/vhl/know-more-about-homeopathy/hahnemann-quotes/

Samuel Hahneman, Organon of Medicine, http://drcherylkasdorf.com/wp-content/uploads/2017/01/Organon-of-Medicine-6th-edition.pdf

Samuel Hahnemann, "Letter to Hering" http://homeoint.org/books4/bradford/chapter68.htm

Steven Decker, Patty Smith and Rudi Varspoor. "The Dynamic Nature of Disease", Chronic Disease in Dr. Hahnemann's Medical System. Page 17

Samuel Hahnemann, Chronic Diseases and Their Cure, translation by S.R. Decker, electronic version

Steven Decker, Patty Smith and Rudi Varspoor. "The Dynamic Nature of Disease", Chronic Disease in Dr. Hahnemann's Medical System. P18

Steven Decker, Patty Smith and Rudi Varspoor. "The Problem", Chronic Disease in Dr. Hahnemann's Medical System. P14

Wikipidea "Chemoreceptor", https://en.wikipedia.org/wiki/Chemoreceptor

Wikipedia. "Élie Metchnikoff", https://en.wikipedia.org/wiki/Élie_Metchnikoff

Wikipedia. "Homoeopathy", https://en.wikipedia.org/wiki/Homeopathy

Wikipedia. "Thalamus". https://en.wikipedia.org/wiki/Thalamus

Wikipedia. "Hypothalamic–pituitary–adrenal axis". https://en.wikipedia.org/wiki/Hypothalamic–pituitary–adrenal_axis

Wikipedia. "Ibuprufen", https://en.wikipedia.org/wiki/Ibuprofen

Wikipedia. "Silicosis". https://en.wikipedia.org/wiki/Silicosis

Wikipedia. "Vitalism". https://en.wikipedia.org/wiki/Vitalism

Yogesh Shegal, "Revolutionized Homeopathy: Sehgal Method of Homoeopathy by Mind". https://www.homeopathy360.com/2018/02/24/revolutionized-homeopathy-sehgal-method-of-homoeopathy-by-mind/

www.ingramcontent.com/pod-product-compliance
Lightning Source LLC
Chambersburg PA
CBHW040314220526
45473CB00009B/2431